BIOENERGY

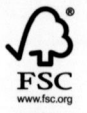

Irene Zweifel-Lanz

BIOENERGY
Understanding the Language of Life

Translated by Aaron Epstein

*To my grandson Severin,
who, with childlike curiosity,
became interested in bioenergetic phenomena
in early childhood and, thanks to that,
taught me a few things.*

Bibliographical Information of the Deutsche Nationalbibliothek
This publication is listed in the Deutsche Nationalbibliographie
of the Deutsche Nationalbibliothek;
detailed bibliographical information can be accessed
under http: //dnb.d-nb.de

© 2016 Irene Zweifel-Lanz

This book was originally published in German under the title
Was ist Bioenergie? by Literareon im Herbert Utz Verlag GmbH.
© 2011 Irene Zweifel-Lanz

Printing, Production and Layout:
BoD – Books on Demand, Norderstedt

ISBN: 978-3-7386-9246-4

TABLE OF CONTENTS

INTRODUCTION 9

1. FOREWORD. 11

2. RETROSPECT AND ACKNOWLEDGMENTS 13

3. BIOENERGY. 16
   3.1 Fundamental notions 16
   3.2 An overview of the characteristics
       of bioenergy 20
       3.2.1 Tradition. 20
       3.2.2 Theory and analogy 25
       3.2.3 Experience and practice. 26
   3.3 Bioenergy today. 29

4. THE PROVABILITY OF BIOENERGY 32
   4.1 Testing bioenergy 32
   4.2 The Tensor 36
       4.2.1 Description of the instrument. 36
       4.2.2 How it can be used 38
   4.3 The three kinds of tests. 39
       4.3.1 Direct testing. 39
       4.3.2 Concentrative testing 41
       4.3.3 Mental testing 41
   4.4 Reproducibility 42

5. BIOENERGETICS OF THE EARTH: GEOPATHY AND GEO-
   MANCY. 45
   5.1 Preliminary remarks. 45
   5.2 The geopathic atmosphere 47
   5.3 Ley lines and vortices 51

6. THE EARTH AS AN ORGANISM 56
   6.1 The fundamental interconnectedness 56
   6.2 The meaning, types, and consequences
       of the interaction between geopathic
       and geomantic phenomena 57
   6.3 Geopathy and geomancy as consciously
       experienced resonance 65

7. THE UNDERSTANDING OF LIFE – RESONANCE,
   INFORMATION, COMMUNICATION 67

8. WATER – THE ENERGETIC PROPERTIES OF
   THE MOST IMPORTANT ELEMENT OF LIFE 75
   8.1 Water is life. 75
   8.2 The repository of vibrations: material and energetic particularities of water. 77
   8.3 Vibrational qualities of water 82
   8.4 Perspective 84

9. BIOENERGY IN HEALING. 88
   9.1 Ancient roots, ancient knowledge. 88
   9.2 The Hippocratic healing tradition 89
   9.3 Different European healing traditions up to
       the middle of the 19th century 90
   9.4 Practical model application of synchronous therapy
       using the Tensor and BIOSYN device 94
       9.4.1 General description of the treatment. 94
       9.4.2 Water treatment. 102
       9.4.3 Isopathic application. 104
       9.4.4 Harmonizing vibrations for the dying process. 105
   9.5 Summary 106

10. CONCLUSION 109

ACKNOWLEDGMENTS 111

ENDNOTES.. 112

FURTHER LITERATURE 117

ABOUT THE AUTHOR 121

INTRODUCTION

What could bring an orthodox medical practitioner – or more precisely, a surgeon and experimental scientist – to write a foreword to a book about bioenergy?

The mundane, material answer is that bioenergy and its related method of healing freed me nearly completely from constant headaches, varying only in their intensity, which had accompanied me for over 40 years. Somewhat less mundane is the answer that orthodox medical practitioners are also aware that there are limits to what can be measured, and that "non-measurability" is not synonymous with "does not exist." Every classical doctor has encountered cases in which both healing and resistance to healing cannot really be explained with our methods, and the wiser among us understand these phenomena, to the benefit of our patients, somewhat sooner. As a veterinarian and experimental researcher, I have long since learned, alongside objective results, to allow space for intuition and, according to circumstances, to trust its guidance. Energy is the basis for every cellular function; without it, no life would be possible. Since energy is not really tangible and confinable to a bottle, the thought itself suggests that energy is something that goes beyond the single cell, and thus also beyond our own limits, that everything in and around us is flowing, and that we are part of a whole.

To extend the answer to the more subtle dimension: Resonance is an important word in both science and in our own lives. No scientist gets good results in a tension-laden environment, just as life in the personal sphere can't go well in such circumstances. Daily interaction with animals as patients – but also as important and inalienable members of the family – reveals in all its urgency the necessity of this vibrational resonance among all us different species of living beings, with nature around us and with other human beings. Not just that we need this resonance in order to be able to communicate with our animals; animals themselves are like resonating bodies and reflect back the vibrations that emanate from ourselves, true to life and unfiltered, as in a mirror. Throughout my life, I have let myself be led by my four-legged companions and their vibrational environment, and I have learned from them to perceive things and atmospheres that would have otherwise remained hidden to me at the intellectual and feeling levels.

From my dogs and cats, I learned to recognize my own positive and negative energies; while my Arabian horses taught me to expand my perceptual horizon with them from "straight ahead" to nearly 360° into the surrounding environment. They also taught me how harmonious movement and rapport – or simply being with them – can be healing for the body and soul while riding, in the same way that watching their wonderfully aesthetic bodies in the meadow can be. They showed me that these vibrations are essential for my life and indispensable to my soul. They are what makes it possible for me to be successful in classical, experimental medicine as well.

Orthodox medicine and bioenergy are thus not mutually exclusive; together, they are an ideal complement to each other. The refreshingly clear words of this book show beyond doubt that here, as well, communication is urgently needed and possible. The author's immense experience and knowledge in the related fields of medicine, physics, and cultural history reflect her lifelong commitment and perseverance.

Brigitte von Rechenberg
Prof. Dr. med. vet. Dipl. ECVS
Zurich, February 2010

> "Reflection is the courage to put up for question the truth of one's own presuppositions and the space of one's own goals."
> Martin Heidegger, *Off the Beaten Track*

1. FOREWORD

North foehn wind in Maloja, Switzerland. Swirling snowflakes – in the glistening sun they resemble a ballet of crystals. Is it not nearly a miracle that each snowflake is said to have its own individual vibrational field and its own unique crystalline structure? Each snowflake is one of a kind. A miracle? What is not reproducible is not scientific, but uniqueness seems to be a characteristic of life.

I would like to invite my readers to reflect and call into question, to research and to test. On the basis of many years of personal experience, in which I have been able to gather data, develop hypotheses, test and apply them in collaboration with a group of interested people, I describe and explain bioenergetic phenomena. This book was requested by clients and seminar participants and inspired by the intelligent and critical questions they asked, as well as innumerable conversations and discussions with family and friends. It is an attempt to (re-)awaken our sensitivity, receptivity or quite simply, curiosity for subtle energy – for the energy which life is made of and which, in what follows, I will call bioenergy.

Precisely because testing and description of bioenergetic phenomena have not stood up to strict scientific criteria until now, a systematic, bioenergetic testing method for making bioenergy visible and a therapeutic approach derived from it are of central importance. Researchers like Masaru Emoto and Fritz-Albert Popp, for example, have had to content themselves until now with "just making bioenergy visible." It may be part of the very nature of bioenergy that, due to its subtle quality, it remains elusive to science.

Personal accounts will enliven and illustrate my text in some chapters. I would like to enable you, dear Reader, to share in my rediscovery and reworking of the ancient knowledge of subtle energy and its integration into a new, holistic worldview.

Since I have always worked independently of the tendencies in vogue, the literature listed in the appendix represents only a limited selection of the works that have enriched me on my path and do not claim to be exhaustive with respect to the subjects treated.

To everyone just becoming acquainted with the subject, and to everyone who has already had personal experience in the area – in short, to all inquiring minds – I wish you interesting discoveries while reading.

Irene Zweifel-Lanz,
Summer 2010

> "People where you live," the little prince said,
> "grow five thousand roses in one garden ...
> yet they don't find what they're looking for... [...]
> And yet what they're looking for could be found
> in a single rose, or a little water..."
> Antoine de Saint-Exupery, *The Little Prince*

2. RETROSPECT AND ACKNOWLEDGMENTS

In 1983, doctor Elisabeth Kapovits from Bielefeld, Germany; teacher and naturopath Angela Paffrath from Kirchzarten, Germany; and electrical engineer Norbert Seiler from Kriens, Switzerland met during a course on bioplasma research given by doctor and author Josef Oberbach. From then on, as a team and full of pioneering spirit, they began to systematically research, test, apply, and disseminate knowledge about bioenergy.

Following studies with Franz Morell, inventor of a pioneering bioresonance device named after him (the Mora device), and drawing upon his own experience and research, Norbert Seiler created a bioresonance device he considered to be more consistent: the BIOSYN device. In addition, with the encouragement of Josef Oberbach, considered to be the "father" of the single-hand spring rod known as the Tensor, he developed a non-technical testing device, the BIONIK Tensor, which he also optimized through extensive experiments of his own.

Although technology in the fields of electrical engineering and electronics had been acquiring increasing importance in bioresonance therapy, Seiler remained true to his original conviction that resonance therapy should rely less on technical refinements and be oriented more directly toward the living person. In this way, energy tests were carried out by this group of like-minded people exclusively with the BIONIK Tensor, and Seiler's BIOSYN device was correspondingly made use of. At the time, this device still functioned according to analog technology.

Over the years, Elisabeth Kapovits, Angela Paffrath, and Norbert Seiler developed courses for systematic testing of bioenergetic phenomena in both the human body and in nature. These courses were given at the time in Kirchzarten and Bielefeld, Germany. The basic courses were addressed to laypeople interested in understanding bioenergy, the advanced courses to people engaged in medical professions.

These three pioneers consciously concentrated on so-called "direct" testing (see Chapter 5.3.1). In this way, they set themselves apart from the esoteric New Age scene that was appearing at the time and, thanks to the systematic approach of "direct" testing, quickly awakened interest and understanding not only in mainstream medicine, but also – and particularly – in pedagogical and theological circles.

For decades, Norbert Seiler was also engaged in intensive studies of the energetic properties of water, particularly in the German study group of Johann Tikale (Igelsbach, Germany). Seiler worked on experiments with molds at Konstanz University on the subject of water quality. Around 1960, he recorded test results in Tikale's group that until today, over 50 years later, have not yet been mentioned in the relevant literature. Seiler's insights into the properties of water represent an important foundation for the fundamental understanding of bioenergy, as well as the therapeutic approach made possible by the biophysical wave and information therapy using the BIOSYN device he developed.

People are led by curiosity, amazement, intuition, personal concern, being deeply moved, and respect to set out on the path toward the great things of life – to the place where the secrets of life are slumbering, the place where the seemingly inexplicable and unsayable await explanation. A few years ago, a handful of people set out on this path with the goal of cultivating and further developing the knowledge passed on by Norbert Seiler.[2] We have dedicated ourselves to the investigation of bioenergy and the responsible dissemination of knowledge on the subject, as well as its application for the benefit of humanity, animals, and plants. Our conviction is that in the places, according to current scientific research, where the boundaries between energy and matter are blurred, the secrets of life are to be found – secrets that have been accessible to pragmatic use and experience since time immemorial.

We wish to make a contribution by supplying the experiences of millennia and (conscious and unconscious) bioenergetic applications with a greater number of verifiable insights. We are continuously calling well-known bioenergetic test and therapeutic procedures into question – not least in order to be able to further develop and optimize our own procedures. In this way, a new generation of devices derived from Norbert Seiler's user device has been developed with a modern electronic configuration and protection from external pollutants.

We would like to thank Elisabeth Kapovits, Angela Paffrath, and Norbert Seiler for their courage in investigating the foundations of the field of subtle energies, unnoticed as it was at the time in academic circles. This was, in fact, the investigation of the very energies that constitute life! We thank them for the knowledge and experience they have left to us as their legacy. It is for us a joy and duty to cultivate and further develop the knowledge we have received.

*"The world of Dasein is a with-world [Mitwelt].
Being-in is Being-with Others. Their Being-in-themselves
within-the-world is Dasein-with [Mitdasein]."*
Martin Heidegger, Being and Time

3. BIOENERGY

3.1 Fundamental notions

Bioenergy is usually defined as subtle energy with life information. We like to relate the term "bioenergy" to the above citation of Martin Heidegger in order to make clear in advance that bioenergy has nothing to do with the physical definition of the concept of energy. In different passages from his writings, the Greek philosopher Aristotle (384-322 B.C.) provides us with the somewhat simplified but, for an understanding of the essence of bioenergy, useful statement that energy is the truly being, and form the possibly being.[3] Renowned research scientists, above all Albert Einstein and Max Planck, came to the conclusion in the course of their investigations that matter as such does not exist, and that matter is a concentration of vibrations in the smallest space. Thus vibrations are among the most fundamental characteristics of all beings. (Vibration is here defined as movement appearing in a regularly recurring, temporal interval.)

Put more simply: Form is condensed energy. The inverse line of reasoning is less familiar: that consequently, without energy there would be no form and therefore no material body. Without the existence of a soul, which doubtless belongs to the area of subtle energy, no living body would be manifest.

Inevitably, the philosophical subject of **Being** and **Appearing**, or of **Having** and **Being** in Martin Buber's sense, suggests itself (Buber, M., (1973). *Das dialogische Prinzip*. Verlag Lambert Schneider GmbH Heidelberg).

Many great authors and poets, initially and particularly those of Spain's baroque age, the so-called "Golden Age," made the subject of being and appearing their subject above all others, anticipating (knowing?) in their poetry and writings that behind the misleading ostensible form, behind the real world, there is a form-building force – an energy. In this way, a large number of poets and philosophers such as Heidegger have dealt in their own way, whether they intended to or not, with bioenergy – with the vibrational patterns and the bioenergetic fields that give form to our life and our world.

For centuries, people were kept at a distance from true esoteric knowledge (Greek εσώτερος [esoteros] = directed inward). Only the initiated and rulers had access to knowledge of the subtle energies. In our current Age of Aquarius – as it is related in books of wisdom and prophecies – ancient knowledge is to be discovered anew, and genuine esoteric knowledge made accessible to all who desire it. But at what price? Each person must be aware that he is today able ("uncalled" and "uninitiated," it is true) to arrive at knowledge that had previously been considered secret – to knowledge that in earlier times, according to ancient laws, he was not entitled to. Dealing with such knowledge must – probably in contrast to earlier times – be learned and integrated as one's own responsibility. Each person who, though "uninitiated," is given the possibility of receiving ancient knowledge, should be aware of the great responsibility that comes along with receiving such knowledge.

Martin Heidegger, in his citation at the beginning of this chapter, may in his own way be giving expression to this responsibility – also in relation to bioenergetic fields: He anticipates, philosophically, the modern-day themes of "information" and "being networked." Speaking about bioenergy without including the keywords "information" and "being networked" is just as meaningless as speaking about information and being networked without having any idea what bioenergy is.

Atoms, cells, organs, and systems such as water, plants, animals, and humans vibrate in their own different, individually typical ways. Greek philosophers from the circle of Heraclitus already pointed to the fact that living systems are open systems in constant interaction with each other. (Cf. the well-known Greek expression πάντα ῥεῖ [panta rhei] = everything flows, said to originate from the circle of the Greek philosopher Heraclitus.)

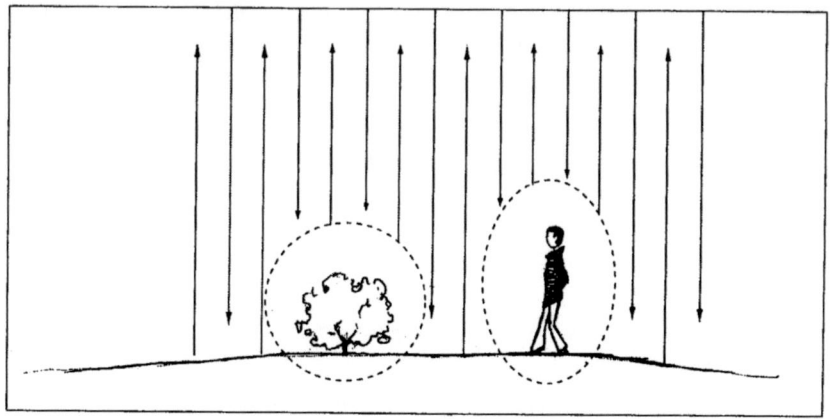

Figure 1: Aura – plants, animals, and humans are open, dissipative systems.
(Illustration: Jacques Laesser)

From the viewpoint of modern physics as well, living systems (plants, animals, and humans) are open and dissipative: Everything is in relationship to everything, or expressed in more modern terms, **everything is networked**. Life is communication. And communication only takes place where networking through bioenergetic fields is present.

If we take as our basis the threefold body-soul-spirit in man, bioenergy is to be found at the juncture between body and soul. It encompasses the preforming patterns, the vital and shaping forces. For this reason, our well-being and mood, health and illness are directly connected with this shining, luminous force of the body and soul.

This is the reason why it is possible, through bioenergetically oriented, therapeutic measures, to have a positive influence on the will and psyche in moments of grief, depression, and other emotionally difficult situations (e.g. exams).

In principle, the vibrational field of bioenergy can be ordered, rhythmic, or harmonious, in which case it is helpful, strengthening, and uplifting. But it may also be unordered, disharmonious, and disintegrating, in which case it has a weakening effect, even draining one to the point of promoting illness.

A bioenergetic vibrational field can also be lacking, or form a so-called zero field, which drains the vitality of the corresponding energy body.

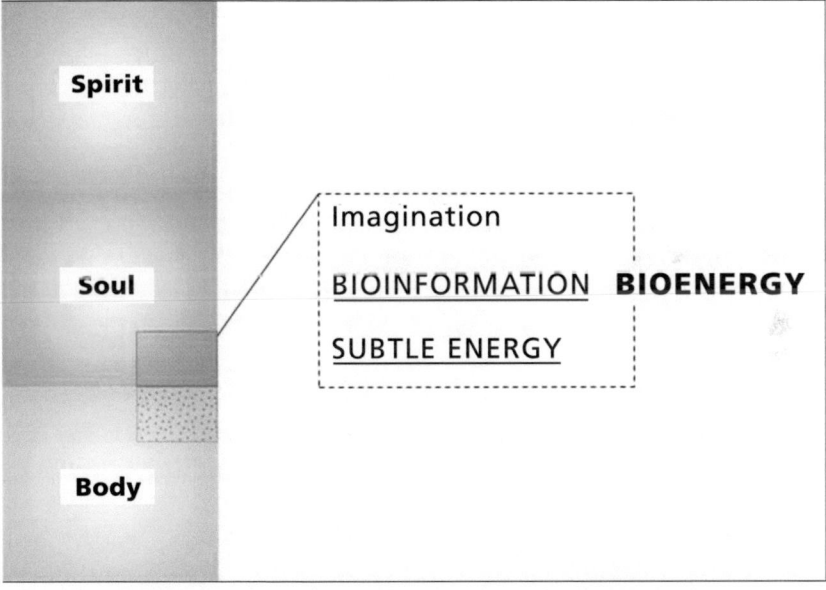

Figure 2: Spirit, soul, body. (Illustration: BIONIK AG)

3.2 An overview of the characteristics of bioenergy

3.2.1 Tradition

The polar life energy, with the components plus and minus (yin and yang) that we call bioenergy, manifests itself throughout the world in sacred and religious buildings, as well as in places of healing and power. In Taoism and acupuncture it is known as chi and, according to the cultural background in question, is also referred to as vital energy, prana, galama, entelechy, od, forming forces, and so on.

Knowledge of this energy was already used in the earliest times, for example to find water and mineral resources. In addition, it formed the basis for healing methods, customs, rituals, and ceremonies.

One of the most impressive examples of the use of bioenergetic knowledge in our Western cultural milieu can be seen in the complex of Epidaurus on the Peloponnesian Peninsula in Greece. To this day it is still possible to experience and test the brilliant collaboration of architects, priests, and doctors. Knowledge of the intertwining of different subtle energetic fields seems to have been internalized at the time. Those who knew certainly sought out the location for this healing center. The theater, which served therapeutic purposes in ancient Greece and was for this reason erected directly beside the therapy building, is located – hardly by chance – on a crossing of powerful ley lines.

The theater of Epidaurus is world-renowned for its unique acoustics. If we analyze this extraordinary phenomenon with bioenergetic knowledge, it turns out that while declaiming, the entire body energy is concentrated on the throat chakra[4], which is responsible for language. In the listener, however, the body energy is concentrated on the ears. The theater is probably also dimensioned with great geometric knowledge. Through it the production of an echo is avoided, firstly since sound waves only reach self-resonance values far behind the spectator room, and secondly, because due to the height of the logarithmically arranged seating rows, all spectators can hear equally well. The actor can thus perform at a normal volume. This also means that bioenergetic phenomena can not only be felt and tested, but also, as in this case, **explained**. For the Romans arriving later, the theater was too small. They constructed a few additional seating rows, but the ingenious system of sound wave transference no longer works for these rows.

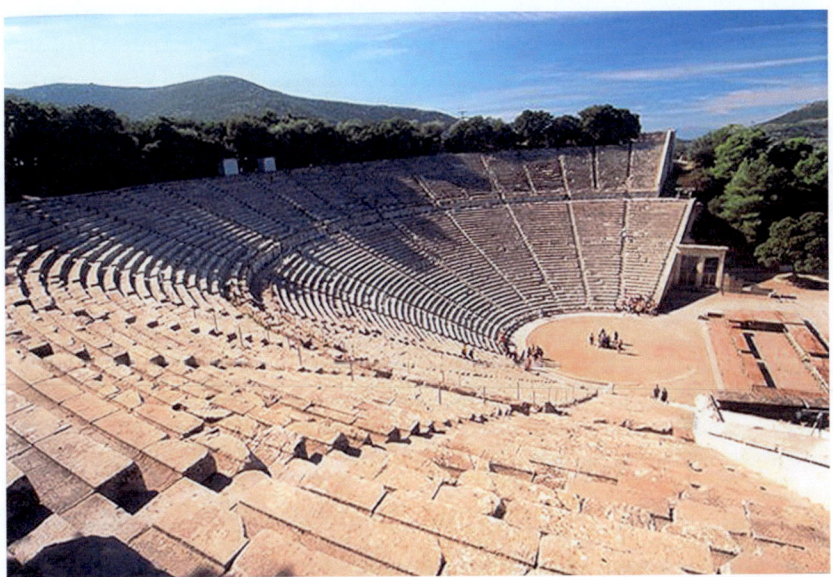

Figure 3: Epidaurus – the original seating sections, built with knowledge of bioenergy, are visible, as well as the sections built later by the Romans. (Photo: Silvia Pfisterer)

Architects' bioenergetic knowledge also included the awareness that dome structures, through particularly strong ground radiation, provide a sort of feedback. Dome constructions are frequently found among ancient advanced civilizations. In later ancient Greece, springs in sanctuaries with dome structures were apparently not simply being covered or protected;

their energy was intentionally potentiated by architectural means. Mosques are also often constructed according to the same principle. The renowned landmark that is the Vatican is most likely the largest dome construction in the world.

Bioenergetic knowledge was present among all ancient peoples to a more or less conscious and more or less cultivated degree. Still today, the sand paintings of the Navajo Indians testify to a traditional, conscious approach to bioenergetic phenomena. Sand paintings are ritual pictures placed on the ground using stones, shells, feathers, etc., according to particular arrangements that energetically support each component of a ceremony. With the preparation and destruction of the sand paintings, the corresponding bioenergetic field is created anew for each ceremonial act.

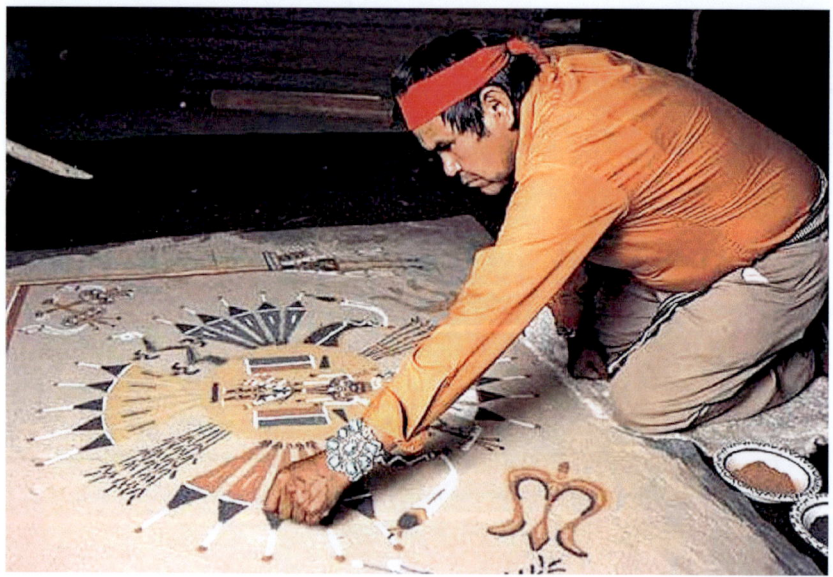

Figure 4: Navajo sand painting.

An example of an intentionally created bioenergetic zero field (lack of subtle energy) is Saint Catherine's Monastery in Sinai, Egypt. Together with the monks' apparent withdrawal into the bleak solitude of the rocky Sinai mountains, the bioenergetically sensitive person finds the non-apparent, but no doubt architecturally consciously created zero field belt, about twenty meters wide around the monastery walls. The monastery is thus not only geographically but also subtle energetically withdrawn from the worldly and cut off from it through an invisible, energetically neutral belt.

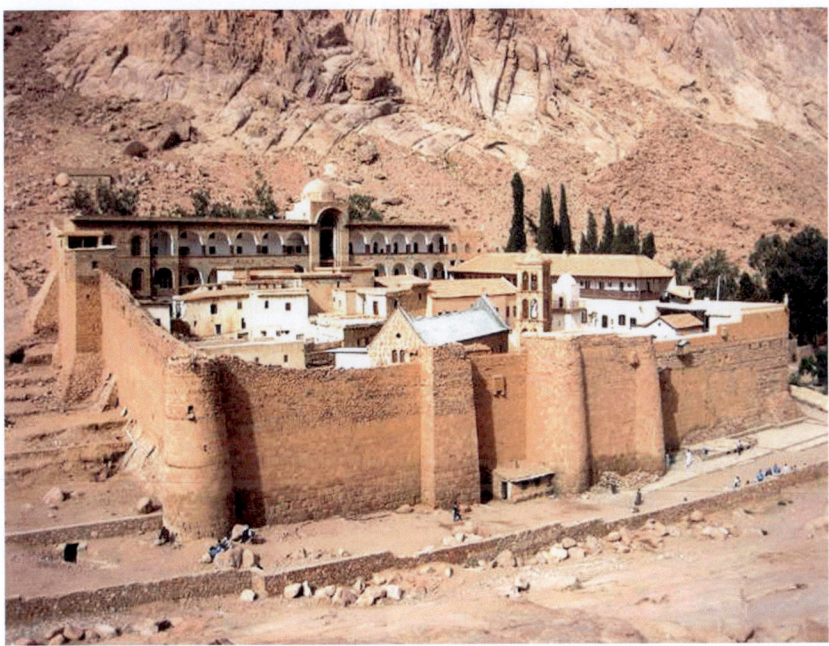

Figure 5: Sinai Monastery – the walls of Saint Catherine's Monastery, surrounded by the invisible yet testable, energetically neutral belt (zero field).

It is revealed above all in religious portrayals that in the Middle Ages bioenergetic knowledge continued to be present in certain sections of the population (chiefly in religious and, it seems particularly, in Jesuit circles). Different representations of halos, as well as hand and finger positions of the infant Jesus and the later Jesus Christ, demonstrate the subtle energetic knowledge of spiritual artists.

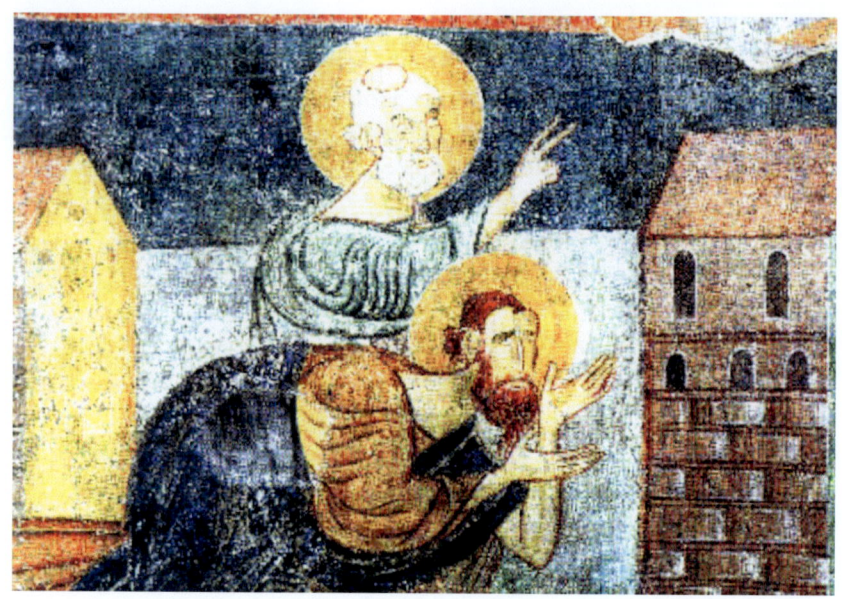

Figure 6: Apostles Peter and Paul – subtle energetically interesting hand position of the Apostles Peter and Paul in prayer and striking representation of the crown chakra of elders/sages. (Photo: Stiftung Pro Kloster St. Johann in Müstair)

For those interested in this area, an ample testing field for using the single-hand spring rod presents itself in museums, for example, in order to gain experience in the field of art and in this way be able to cast a glance behind the scenes.

It is quite well known that this knowledge among the people was prohibited and annihilated with thousands of burnings at the stake. The energetic and thus necessarily holistic worldview was definitively replaced by a mechanistic, rational worldview during the Enlightenment. With René Descartes (1598-1650) and his disciples, the purely intellectual, scientific age was born, in which the ancient fundamental, holistic experiential knowledge of subtle energies and working with them no longer had any place, since according to the new scientific criteria, it was neither provable nor comprehensible. Extremely ancient knowledge was sacrificed to the flames, and despite being passed down orally, was lost over time. Interestingly, the powerful of this world always knew about bioenergetic phenomena or were at least surrounded by advisers who were initiated into subtle energetic knowledge (cf. 8.3).

3.2.2 Theory and analogy

Today's science, particularly the still relatively young elementary particle physics, is acquiring more and more knowledge that directly, or through analogy, leads to an understanding of bioenergy.

Particularly impressive is the atomic model of Louis de Broglie (1892-1987). It states that each atom, molecule, and system has its own typical wave field. Healthy systems have stable, ordered field patterns. Systems that are ill have chaotic, disintegrating fields. De Broglie is here describing scientifically the same subtle energetic conditions that we can comprehend and describe with what is considered as unscientific – the single-hand spring rod.

A highly controversial statement is made by the so-called Einstein-Podalski-Rosenstein-Paradox[5] which proves that split subatomic particles have an effect on one another, even when they are flying away from each other at more than the speed of light.

The English biologist Rupert Sheldrake (born 1942) created a revolution in the scientific worldview by developing the model of morphogenetic fields, which store the information and experiences of life. He approaches here the ancient Indian knowledge of the Akashic Records: All and everything is already present on an informational level. Corresponding information and energies can be collected from the information pool at any time (cf. 3.3, p.15 and Sheldrake, R., (1983). *A New Science of Life: the hypothesis of formative causation*, Los Angeles, CA: J.P. Tarcher, 1981).

Fritz-Albert Popp (born 1938, postdoctoral qualification in theoretical radiology and biophysics) investigated the radiation of living cells and proved that it is measurable as ultraweak coherent light. With the light intensifier he constructed, Popp showed that cells communicate with each other through so-called biophotons. Their activity is the measure of vitality, for example, of food. Cancer cells, in contrast, do not communicate and do not radiate light any longer. Unfortunately, cancer research has thus far been unable to profit from this knowledge. (Popp, F. A., (1999). *Die Botschaft unserer Nahrung.* Verlag Zweitausendundeins, Frankfurt.)

Until this day, bioenergy is measurable above all through its action, as is also the case with magnetism. Indirect and pictorial interpretations are possible with Kirlian and crystallization photography, the Steigbild and Drop Picture methods, as well as through measurement of change in bodily resistance, special low-frequency spectrum analysis, etc. Making bioenergetic phenomena visible is, one must say, something quite impressive. In this area we owe much to Popp and his development of the light intensifier, and the St. Petersburg physicist Konstantin Korotkov with his further development of Kirlian photography.[6] These results are still not considered sufficient for university science.

3.2.3 Experience and practice

Because plants, animals, and humans are open systems that are in a so-called steady state, bioenergy is fundamentally perceptible to each person to a more or less intensive degree. We often deal with bioenergy in our everyday lives unconsciously or as a vague feeling. Bioenergy can be physically experienced by anyone by means of the kinesiological muscle test.[7] Bioenergy can be applied as a complementary method of healing in biocybernetics, bioresonance therapy, magnetic field therapy, kinesiology, acupuncture, acupressure, polarity, and other fields. Every healthy person can, with some practice, systematically test and make bioenergy visible with the single-hand spring rod.

In most people, the quality of bioenergy is perceived through changes in sensitivity in the somatic, psychological area. People with some practice are familiar with the "numb feeling" that is felt in a bioenergetic zero field and have experienced yawning during global earthquakes, during which the bioenergy is disturbed for hours and people become tired. Everyone interested can experience the positive and negative effects of bioenergy when they allow it to act on them in natural surroundings or at sacred places and vortices, monasteries, and churches.

Animals and plants also react with great sensitivity to subtle energies. They are hardly influenceable, and for this reason they are more credible in many situations than the doubting human being, calling everything critically into question.

We have carried out the following experiment several times: We placed two different drinking bowls in front of sick animals – one with normal tap water, the other with individually tested healing water. Until now there has not been a single sick animal that has not spontaneously chosen the bowl with healing water. We also had animal owners repeat the experiment.

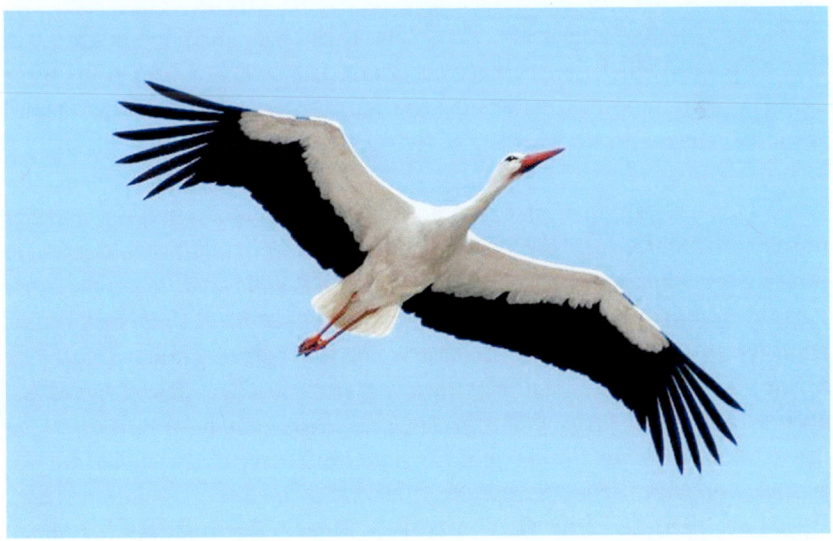

Figure 7: Stork – stork wings act like bioenergetic antennas.

Storks, whose wings look like antennas, like to settle on houses with good bioenergy. Probably for this reason they often sought out churches before church towers started being equipped with mobile phone antennas. One year after the church in Kirchzarten, Germany, was energetically refurbished, the storks – who had been absent for years – moved in again, definitively. We can assume that the widespread image of storks as bringers of babies is also related to the fact that in a bioenergetically healthy house where storks were nesting, there would be blessings for the children as well. The connection between difficult pregnancies, miscarriages, or even infertility in houses that are poorly supplied energetically is generally known today to those working in the area of subtle energy.

The sensitivity with which plants react to subtle energies can be experienced by any plant friend when he tries placing a poorly growing plant in another location, perhaps also placing it beside a different neighboring plant, and testing the type and quantity of fertilizer, as well as the water quantity needed by the plant. Interesting phenomena in this connection are reported by Peter Tomkins and Christopher Bird in "The Secret Life of Plants" (1973), Harper and Row. One thing they describe is the reaction of plants which let their leaves droop the moment that crabs were being cooked in boiling water next to them: a nice example of the mutual responsiveness and networking of living systems.

For his general qualification examination in Biology, student S.V. presented a study on tomatoes and their bioenergetic behavior in relation to music. He rented a greenhouse in a plant nursery, planted tomato seedlings of the same variety, and for weeks had rock music played to some of them and music from Johann Sebastian Bach to others. The third group grew without any music played to it. The result was amazing: three totally different tomatoes, even with regard to taste, with different-sized leaves and bushes. We had the opportunity to follow the entire study with the Tensor and assigned leaves, bushes, and fruit to the corresponding bushes by means of a relational test. It was energetically clear: Bach was the winner – the tomatoes his music was played to were, without exception, the largest and tastiest, and their foliage the greenest.

3.3 Bioenergy today

As we have seen, bioenergy remains unmeasurable to this day in the strictly scientific sense. Bioenergy – and particularly its action – can, however, be experienced and tested. A tester with a single-hand spring rod can make the quality and quantity of energy visible. Ideally, such tests are repeatable: Different (experienced) testers obtain the same test results when they are sufficiently well practiced, directly test the bioenergy in a strictly systematic way (cf. Chapter 4.3.1), and are not working under stress.

Aristotle believed there had to be a particular form-building force and called this **entelechy** – "that which carries its goal in itself."[8] In the same way, the doctor Paracelsus (1493-1541) recognized the ordering principle and called it **archeus**, that is, "spiritual body." He describes the archeus as, among other things, the immaterial principle that is responsible for health and illness.[9]

At the beginning of the last century, the biologist and philosopher Driesch[10] (1867-1941) understood the processes of life not only through chemistry and physics, but he saw them as also determined by entelechy. His theory, according to which an independent life force determines all life processes, influenced the biologist Alexander Gurwitsch (1874-1954) who, like Driesch before him and Sheldrake after him, spoke of morphogenetic fields, biological fields that he considered to be non-physical. In his later years, Gurwitsch dedicated himself to investigating the information concerning the process of biological structuring that could be gained from these fields.

The term "morphogenetic fields," however, first became well known and a worthy topic of discussion thanks to the English biologist Rupert Sheldrake. Sheldrake is also of the opinion that they are not electromagnetic (that is, physical) fields, describing them instead in the sense of the ancient Indian or Theosophical "Akashic Records": He defines morphogenetic fields – similar to the way the Akashic Records are described – as invisible structures that give the universe shape and form.

According to this view, a field pattern is present behind every structure that is formed for the first time, whether it is a thought, action, or cellular structure – a field pattern that is not of an electromagnetic nature and is beyond space and time. The more often a corresponding structure is formed, the more it strengthens "morphic resonance." Thanks to researchers like Sheldrake and Popp (biophoton research), today we are capable of imagining and recognizing interactions in the exceedingly complex organization of living systems.

Not only adaptation, but forming and cooperation seem to be the basis of life and evolution.

Modern man has to a large extent lost the sensory apparatus for subtle energy. For this reason he is understandably afraid of everything that cannot be proven and explained with scientifically documentable studies and experiments. After reading the reports of researchers like Sheldrake, Popp, Heisenberg (1901-1976), and Capra (born 1939), we can imagine that a new science could indeed be developed, a science that includes the realm of subtle energy. All world cultures except recent Western culture take the existence of an intermediary realm of subtle matter for granted, a realm that possesses both physical and spiritual characteristics.[11]

What is the origin of the sharp contrast up until now between spiritless, soulless matter on the one hand and an immaterial soul or spirit on the other?

Various cultural and historical stages contributed to the effacing and annihilation of the ancient holistic knowledge and making it unprovable. Since the Enlightenment, lines of reasoning have been one-dimensional and linear, that is, limited to what is exclusively material. The Council of Constantinople (869-870) played a decisive role in this regard by condemning the old threefold division of man into body, soul, and spirit. Then, at the latest, the twofold division (dichotomy) of body and soul was introduced, the spiritual here being ascribed to the soul and thus losing its independent status. This was a debasement of the spiritual, which was then confused with the psychological, which actually belongs to the domain of the soul. In the end, this process led to the Cartesian dualism between coarse matter (body) as "res extens" and spirit as "res cogitans." Here began the unfortunate confusion of spirit and mind. This is a dualism that would culminate in the total abandonment of the spirit, leaving behind coarse matter as the only reality. Thus science, with all its knowledge as a boon and benefit to man, could develop – but fatally, as everything from the subtle energetic domain was considered **not calculable, not measurable**, suspicious, and thus not integrated into conventional knowledge.

The time is ripe for the nature and action of the subtle life energy that we call bioenergy to be recognized once again and for us to be able to employ it consciously in our everyday lives, as well as in the most varied professional and other domains, in order to improve our quality of life.

We are led to rediscover the quality of the nature of bioenergy and its means of action by the terms information, communication, and resonance. Bioenergetic phenomena are, by definition, phenomena of resonance. **And: Resonance always has to do with information and communication.**

After this assessment of bioenergy today, the practical approach is the following:

- How can bioenergy be tested and made visible and useful in everyday life?
- How can scientific results and statements be compared, if necessary, with our test results?
- How can we strive toward and realize a mutually fruitful exchange of ideas between different disciplines?
- How could knowledge about subtle energy serve science by enriching and promoting it?
- How can science possibly promote the understanding of subtle energies?

> "What we know is a drop,
> what we don't know is an ocean."
> Isaac Newton

4. THE PROVABILITY OF BIOENERGY

4.1 Testing bioenergy

Radiesthesia (as the field of vibrational divination is called, Lat. radius = ray) is, generally speaking, the technical term for the teaching that detects and assesses the action of radiation emitted from living or nonliving objects, living beings, the cosmos, and the earth. This action can be detected by sensitive people with dowsing rods or pendulums, and by any healthy person trained accordingly with the Tensor (cf. 4.2.-4.4.). Already in the Middle Ages, what we refer to as "testing bioenergy" was called radiesthesia. Radiesthesia was carried out by sensitive people – radiesthetists – usually with a pendulum or dowsing rod.

In all ancient cultures there were people with knowledge who were able to test radiation of all types in one way or another and also did this, for example, for the village community (the Indians) or for sacred communities (the Celts). The fact that radiesthesia (or dowsing) acquired a bad reputation is related firstly to a lack of understanding of subtle energies and secondly to abuses and charlatanism, as well as rejection by the church. In a decree of the Vatican in 1924, the church granted permission to dowsers for the purposes of searching for springs and investigating sleeping locations. For all other activities, the dowsing rod was the work of the devil. Today in Switzerland, however, there is an association for radiesthesia and geobiology once again.[12]

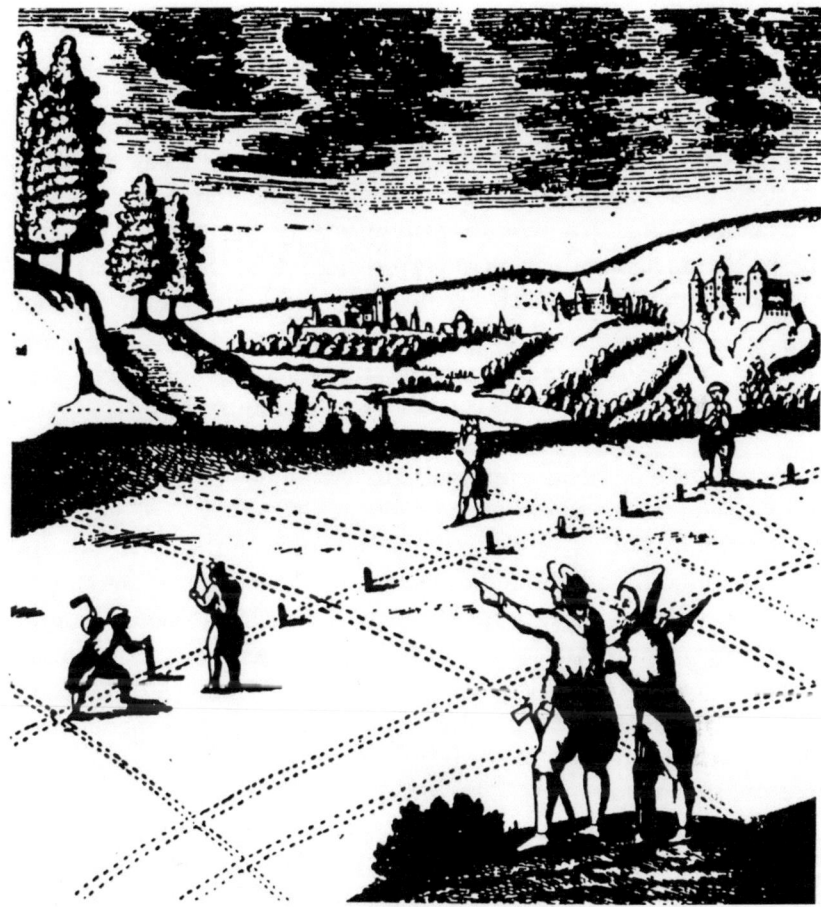

Figure 8: Dowsing rod – search for ore veins by means of a dowsing rod.
(From: Roessler "Speculum metallurgicum politissimum" 1700)

Bioenergy can be tested and felt in many different ways. It is possible to demonstrate the action of bioenergetic phenomena on nerves and muscles by means of different testing devices. In both the kinesiological muscle test and tests using the single- and two-hand spring rods, corresponding nerves are always involved in addition to particular muscle fibers.

With a defined and systematic approach, bioenergy can be tested and made visible and experienceable quite objectively. If Popp with his light intensifier is able to differentiate between foods according to their corresponding exchange of biophotons, then with the single-hand spring rod we have the possibility, in the simplest and quickest way, of making precisely these bioenergetic differences visible and understandable to us personally. Cellular communication is bioenergy. The vibration made visible by the single-hand spring rod is produced due to the intensity of the ultracoherent light radiated by the biophotons: the stronger the radiation, the stronger the light, and the greater the amplitude of the testing device. In other words: the more intensive the amplitude, the more intensive the cellular communication. **Life is (cellular) communication.**

If Snow White had had a bioenergetic testing device, she would have recognized that the beautiful red apple was dangerous and would not have eaten it. With a single-hand spring rod and the corresponding training, foods can be tested for their digestibility and differentiated from foods that merely fill one's stomach – a possibility that is becoming increasingly significant for the future of our diet. We can test foods, eyeglasses, jewelry, medications, teas, and many other items by ourselves, freed from labels, publicity-promoted foods and medications, diets, and nutritional plans. Testing should not make us dependent, but **free and independent**. Specific, personal intolerances can also be tested for therapeutic purposes.

Bioenergy is the hidden reality, so to speak; but we have to a large extent lost the sensory apparatus to perceive it. A beautiful red apple is not necessarily an energetically good apple beneficial to our health. Not just in fairy tales are beautiful red apples poisoned. As people who have grown up in the materialistic age, we nevertheless do have the tendency to reach for the red apple, rather than the one with spots…

It is a matter of importance to us to convey and teach the so-called "direct testing," so as to avoid as much mysticism as possible and to establish new models of explanation. This has brought us, at least in "open" scientific circles, a certain degree of acceptance, and in some cases has enabled positive collaboration to take place.

It is worthwhile to learn the skills of direct testing through a clear, understandable system. These testing skills can be learned by any healthy person. In addition, basic knowledge about bioenergy should be acquired in order to understand what is really being tested. Whoever has mastered just the basic skills can already help themselves in their everyday life.

Whoever has a deeper interest in testing atmospheric environments affected by bioenergy – in the narrower and wider senses of the term – should be introduced, theoretically and practically, to the systematic testing of the most important geopathic and geomantic phenomena: Water veins and cosmically and terrestrially aggravated lines (meaning stress for bedrooms!) can also be tested with the help of a clear system. Mental openness is called for in this area, since due to environment-dependent changes or meteorological conditions, sudden energetic imbalances can often manifest.

For those with therapeutic interests, it is important to know that, with the Tensor and the so-called **direct** (not mental) **method of testing**, the human body can be energetically diagnosed. Subtle energetic therapies and applications can also be tested in this way.

The single-hand spring rod is a crutch. By practicing with the Tensor (or a similar instrument and similar method), our inner indicator, our inner, atrophied sensory apparatus for subtle energies develops. There should never be any dependency on a person or instrument. By being independent of today's noisy advertising and fashionable trends of all kinds and in every sector, we acquire more personal responsibility, something that usually brings happiness to a free human spirit.

4.2 The Tensor

4.2.1 Description of the instrument

In order to make manifest their subjective perception, humans have since time immemorial made use of a technique in which they hung an unsteady balance on an object, through which a tension was created that was disturbed by the influence of even the most minute vibrational differences. The most well-known of these is the forked branch, the so-called dowsing rod (German: "Wünschelrute" from Old High German "Wunseiligerda"), which, by bending the two branches in opposite directions with the correct hand position, was set under tension and held in equilibrium in this tension. The wooden handle of the BIONIK Tensor is patterned on this ancient dowsing rod. It offers the advantage, in comparison with other similar instruments, that the tester hardly becomes tired, and the energy flows optimally and harmoniously through the previously tested wood.

The "Tensor" (from Lat. tendere = to stretch out, hold out the hand) is a single-hand spring rod that is suitable for testing subtle energies. As such, it is an indicator for bioenergetic states and bioenergetic phenomena. With the Tensor, according to a well-elaborated system that has proven itself for years, terrestrial and cosmic energetic states, energetic anomalies in landscapes and buildings, and ley lines and vortices can be tested and described according to their respective energetic qualities and quantities.

BIONIK Tensors consist of a wooden handle with a socket at the base for an attachable cable connected to a wooden, bell-shaped receiver (this enables the tester to remain outside of the pathological vibration of a client or medication). The antenna wire is located at the top of the handle, with a disc-shaped ring attached to it. The wire is made of a previously tested alloy that guarantees maximum suppleness with optimum strength.

The Tensor forms, along with the hand and arm, a finely regulated vibrational system. The ring, antenna wire, and handle are attuned to each other in such a way that they are readily set into vibration by the smallest hand movements. The ring is grooved on one side and thus polarized. Due to the polarity differences between men and women, this must be taken into account particularly during polarity tests.

Since lightweight Tensors "waggle" and "whirr," taking in too many foreign energies as a result, a certain weight (primarily the wooden handle with some metal on the inside) was consciously taken into consideration during the development of the BIONIK Tensor. This is especially decisive for the energetic diagnosis of people.

The wood for Tensor handles is tested anew for each production by a woodturner in Schwarzenberg, Switzerland. Beech, cherry, or more recently, plum tree wood is usually chosen. Pear tree wood, for example, is very poor for this purpose, since that type of wood transfers energy to only a moderate degree.

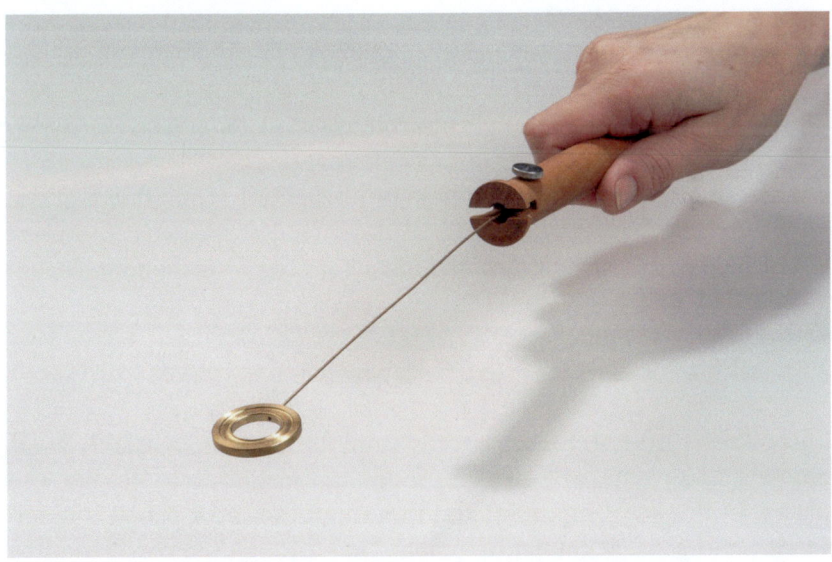

Figure 9: Tensor – the BIONIK Tensor. (Photo: BIONIK AG)

4.2.2 How it can be used

Today there are more and more reasons to become involved in bioenergetic phenomena and perceptions. In a time when our quality of life and our environment are being called into question by increasingly problematic developments, personal responsibility and independent thought and action are becoming ever more important. The inclusion of bioenergy – that is, a finer quality of energy and its possibility of being tested with the Tensor – opens for us the opportunity to better deal with a whole series of current environmental and health problems: for example, by testing the vitality and digestibility of foods, drinks, clothing, locations (bed location, office chair, etc.), glasses, or jewelry. Geopathic and geomantic conditions can also be revealed and changes verified which is becoming more and more important for preserving our health. The current turning point in our times is certainly responsible for the fact that many renowned scientists are becoming seriously interested in this area, which only a few years ago was considered metaphysics, and are providing more and more insights into it.

The amplitude of the Tensor gives us information about whether the bioenergy is
- ordered, rhythmic, and harmonious = beneficial, strengthening, and structuring;
- unordered, disharmonious, and disintegrating = weakening, deconstructing, and
- illness-promoting;
- or lacking and forming a zero field, which drains vitality.

These Tensor indications are equally valid for the human earthly body, animals, and plants, as well as for foods and medications, objects, and places. In this way, important and meaningful tests for people and animals (on organs, acupuncture points, etc.) through the corresponding bioenergetic fields can be made.

With the Tensor, many different kinds of tests can be carried out:

Self-test: Checks the tester's energetic state.
Place test: Checks the energetic characteristics of the test site.
Room test: Geopathic analysis of the site, room.
Energy test: Analysis of the energetic intensity of people, animals, plants, or rooms.
Relational test: Tolerance test (medications, foods, jewelry, body care products, tea varieties, etc.).
Polarity test: With the polarity test, the most subtle determinations of bioenergetic phenomena can be made; it is always complementary to the energy test. Precise determinations of water quality are chiefly made with this test. It is the most difficult one to learn, but offers remarkable possibilities for energetic diagnosis.
Distance test: With corresponding practice and experience, all the tests described above can also be done for the surrounding environment. Thus it is possible, for example, from a suitable location, to test entire landscapes, mountain chains, and forests, and to analyze them accordingly.

4.3 The three kinds of tests

4.3.1 Direct testing

Direct testing with the Tensor is easiest for most people, and for the practiced tester it has few possibilities for error. Direct testing means neutrally recording the vibration or energy field of an object, organ, etc., without innerly posing a question. When this form of testing has been thoroughly learned and practiced, and the preconditions (self-test, place test, global energy situation) are acceptable, no errors appear with the direct energy and relational test, and rarely with the more subtle polarity test.

Polarities are not something that separate, but that connect. Polarity means the uttermost heterogeneity and yet connectedness between the poles; this means that while doing a direct test of polarities, an energy flow manifests between plus and minus. The direct polarity test is more difficult than the energy test. It can also not be carried out with all standard Tensor models. For someone who is well practiced, polarities reveal subtle energetic phenomena in a more differentiated way than an energy test. In addition, during direct testing, the results can be continuously verified with reference to a 1.5 volt tubular battery. Even a fully drained 1.5 volt tubular battery still has a minimal energy field that aids in verification when a difficult global energetic situation appears that could, for example, alter the tester's own energy, thus falsifying the test's interpretation. Plus and minus poles are defined on the tubular battery. Our test results can be verified with reference to these poles as long as the results are within the polar area.

The precondition for direct testing with the Tensor is for the tester to act as a neutral observer without expectations and without desires or conceptions. The subconscious contributes to the synchronization of the device's movement, and the attention is directed through observing the Tensor ring and test object. People trained in the sciences and people who are accustomed to thinking objectively will have access to this testing method most readily. This method is the least fatiguing and, because the bioenergy is directly registered, has a very low rate of error.

Direct testing is the most immediate way of revealing the form and action of energetic phenomena. This type of testing and the practical application of bioenergy help us to experience and understand correlations and interactions between the material and subtle worlds. In this way we have the opportunity of better understanding our environment and our preferences and aversions, as well as ourselves. Direct testing makes enriching insights into interrelations in life possible. We can find and analyze these interrelations ourselves, and we can verify and optimize what we have learned theoretically.

As a result, new aspects of our hobbies, profession, and cultural interests become accessible to us in a new dimension. The disadvantage of the direct testing method is a certain limitation on what is immediately present and the local and wider energetic conditions.

4.3.2 Concentrative testing

Concentrative testing is typical for the dowser who concentrates on a specific vibration, usually water veins. It furthers one's testing possibilities. Through inner concentration, through focusing one's attention on something specific that is to be tested, it is possible to choose one possibility out of many – for example, a particular type of energy, a state, or a sensible therapeutic measure. This form of testing is especially helpful when the energetic sphere is formed of several types of energy, like in a human being, for example, in which the different organs, glands, bodily fluids, and so on contribute to the sum of the entire energy field. When we only test a part of the body directly, it is possible that the result we obtain will refer to the sum of the different energies. As a concentration aid, specific arrangements, checklists, hair, saliva, or other sources of personal vibrations can be helpful. The range of possibilities for ideas has no limits. What is decisive is that we focus on the information.

The role of the subconscious and the outward attention is, with concentrative testing, similar to that of direct testing. Additionally, we consciously focus, innerly, on something specific that must be something known. Here we already encounter the first possibilities of error: errors of concentration, concentrating on something false or on something that does not exist, or lack of knowledge and skills. With direct and concentrative testing, however, it is possible to apprehend energetic phenomena quite precisely and clearly.

4.3.3 Mental testing

With the typical form of mental testing, as it is found most frequently in the use of the pendulum, a question is posed to the subconscious and a preset answer – usually yes/no – is expected. With this somewhat magical form of testing, it is theoretically possible to test everything. It is possible to ignore preconditions that are necessary for the first two kinds of tests, and even to go beyond space and time. If the limits of space and time can be transcended, however, the pendulum user must be aware of his own connection and dependence, his own re-ligio (Lat. religere = reconnect). The turning movement of the pendulum is strongly dependent on the pendulum user's personal attitude and the expression of his will. The most minimal bodily reactions are transferred to the pendulum.

In order to consistently attain a more than 50% accuracy rate in yes/no questions, one must be able to reliably handle one's own consciousness and personal state of health. And precisely here is where the most common sources of error are to be found: lacking or misleading imaginative powers, false questions or false formulations, and unconsciously anticipated answers. Our own subconscious quickly outwits us, and our own state (fatigue, pressure to succeed) or outward conditions lead to testing errors. There tends to be the danger of dealing with energetic phenomena too abstractly and relying too much on the force of imagination, or of getting lost in spiritist realms. It is certainly not for nothing that many great books of wisdom warn against using the pendulum.

We recommend, above all to beginners, to work only with direct testing and possibly later with concentrative testing.

4.4 Reproducibility

Following methodical training and sufficient practice on one's own, and exercising constant self-restraint, it is possible to obtain results with the Tensor that are of high probability and reproducibility. There are, firstly, well-elaborated, standardized rules for testing and interpretation and, secondly, simple testing aids (such as the 1.5 volt tubular battery) in order to provide safeguards for results and enable them to be reproduced by several individuals.

The problem of non-reproducibility is usually not due to the method. In most cases, this is the problem of the tester or people tested. Raimar Banis (born 1951), doctor for naturopathy and general medicine and developer of so-called psychosomatic energetics, experienced himself that the best testers, who could report a 90% success rate in their own practice, only achieved a rate of 50% when they were under pressure and felt compelled to succeed.

We could thus go so far as to characterize direct testing as a "school for life," as a process from incessant (if often unconscious) thinking toward emptiness. It seems to us that we only believe what we see. In reality, it is the other way around: We only see what we believe. This thought is what makes neutral direct testing so difficult, and it was this line of reasoning that enabled Werner Heisenberg, in February 1927, to discover one of the most important laws of quantum physics: the Uncertainty Principle. (Heisenberg, W. *Der Teil und das Ganze*. Munich, 1969). On this subject, we must also accept that the prevailing conditions of society and the scientific enterprise resulting from it were never conducive to developing research in frontier areas.

Each of us can reflect for ourselves on how far the personal challenge of a good tester and of groups that wish to demonstrate reproducibility can go. For science, an experiment must be reproducible, but with living, dissipative systems, this is a priori only conditionally possible, since living, open systems exhibit flowing and moving corpuscles (= energy fields). Scientific reproducibility here often resembles (according to the test object) the attempt to draw the same water twice from a flowing

stream, thus showing a lack of understanding of fundamental bioenergetic knowledge. If we consider that everything in us, all the way to our individual cells, is communication and resonance, it is obvious that every subtle energetic test exhibits a parapsychological aspect.

Similar non-reproducible results to those of radiesthetists have been obtained by clairvoyants and physicians. Nonetheless, Korotkov was able, with his GDV (gas discharge visualization) technique, to measure changes in emotional state and laying on of hands almost immediately through a change in the electromagnetic field. We can also cite Popp's video in this connection, in which the action of healing hands is made visible through the light intensifier. Although we are here treading, whether we wish to or not, at least partially in the parapsychological domain, the lack of intent and avoiding every possible source of interference is eminently important. Strict control of our thoughts, knowledge of our own subconscious and consciousness, inner emptiness, and neutrality toward the test object are the challenge for each and every tester.

In groups, it will probably only be possible to attain reproducibility when the above-mentioned preconditions are set, or when the participants are **testers who trust and have positive attitudes toward each other, are capable of innerly distancing themselves from their everyday life, and do not allow themselves to be brought into "test stress."** It could be advantageous for a group of testers – when the goal is to do experiments for reproducibility – to mutually attune themselves together in, for example, a meditation or ritual, thus placing themselves, subtle energetically speaking, under a common roof. Sabotage programs – usually unconscious – from one's own circle or from observers are not to be underestimated. Our own field must be strong in order to not be influenced by a suspicious observer.

From the results of theoretical and experimental physics, it follows that **after every measurement, what was measured has changed**, and a reality independent of the consciousness of the observer does not exist. Consequently, every act of research, that is, every measurement and observation, represents the creation of a particular (and in each case new) reality. Thus the question presents itself of what significance reproducibility really has in each particular discipline, and of the decisive consequences it does or does not have for subtle energetic tests and applications, and for subtle energetic research in general.

> *"Chi is the structured pattern of relationships, which are defined in a directional way."*
> Fritjof Capra

5. BIOENERGETICS OF THE EARTH: GEOPATHY AND GEOMANCY

5.1 Preliminary remarks

As far as we can trace back in different cultures, the perception of differences in the bioenergetic (= electromagnetic) radiation of the ground from place to place was something that man possessed. According to the cultural milieu, man refined this radiation in order to improve his quality of life, or made use of it, with higher knowledge, for rituals and/or ritual locations. We can go as far back as Moses, who found water with his rod. The capability of perceiving the earth's radiation was suppressed to a greater and greater extent through science and technology and relegated to the realm of the preposterous. Seen as unnecessary and no longer in keeping with our times, these abilities were no longer cultivated, and they atrophied as a result. The corresponding knowledge was no longer passed on, and if it was, then behind closed doors.

Still today, nomads observe where their dogs lie down to sleep, and this is where they set up their own places to sleep. Dogs, like horses and cows, are so-called fleers from radiation, as are people – in contrast to cats and bees, for example, which seek out unsettling energies. Black Elk, the wise man of the Oglala Sioux, describes in his book *Black Elk Speaks* (1932, William Morrow & Company) how, when building a new village, the knowers of his tribe first determined the places for the (sleeping) tents.

It is not as if the modern human organism no longer registers such vibrational differences; rather, most people are no longer conscious of them. A person's body is nonetheless impregnated and informed by the vibrations of the place where he spends his time, above all, while resting. This can be tested on a person through an energetic diagnosis, which often makes it possible to explain sleeping and other disturbances (e.g. inexplicable miscarriages). Animals, for the most part, still have a sensory apparatus for unusual vibrations and energies and naturally avoid places that are not good for them from an energetic point of view.

A dog and his owners recently moved into a beautiful villa. He hadn't touched his large, comfortable dog basket for six weeks, but lay instead on the floor beside it. Underneath the dog basket, we tested a massive terrestrial disturbance line, and we also noticed that the dog basket was lying in front of a mirror, due to which the disturbance line was reflected and thus intensified. We moved the dog basket about 50 centimeters, so that it was no longer affected by the disturbing emissions. In a matter of seconds, the dog lay down in it, right in the middle of the day. He had waited six weeks to finally curl up in his cozy bed.

Healthy horses eat their feed right away and do so very quickly. The horse belonging to a riding teacher attracted attention because he would take a mouthful of feed from his feeding trough, then hastily turn around in a circle in his box, take another mouthful of feed and circle around once more. When the box was tested with the Tensor, a crossing of water veins and terrestrial disturbance lines was revealed in precisely the place where the big animal had to place his legs while feeding. Because of this, he never felt calm while feeding. We harmonized this disturbing vibration and, from one day to the next, the horse began to eat his feed peacefully and rapidly, just like all the other horses.

A woman owned a dog and a cat. After moving into a new house, the cat always lay on the owner's bed, something that seemed suspicious to her, since she was familiar with bioenergetic knowledge. The dog, totally fixated upon the woman, wouldn't go into the bedroom at all, despite being encouraged and pleaded with to do so. Our test provided the verification that the location of the woman's bed was bioenergetically poor, that is, a vibrationally disturbed location for a bed. Since there was no possibility of moving the bed, we attempted to improve the situation energetically. The next day it was reported that the cat was now sleeping in front of the bedroom door and the dog in the bedroom, next to the bed. This is a nice example of the behavior of so-called fleers of radiation and radiation seekers.

5.2 The geopathic atmosphere

The geopathic atmosphere is formed firstly of natural cosmic and terrestrial vibrations and, secondly, is changed through natural causes (for example, meteorological changes) and causes arising from technology and civilization (for example, power lines). The new medical-radiesthetic field of geopathy was founded by the dowser Gustav Freiherr von Pohl who, in the Bavarian city of Visbiliburg, radiesthetically investigated the bed locations of cancer patients and determined that all of them were found in bioenergetically precarious zones. At the time, Pohl held "harmful" and "weakening" earth radiations responsible for the illnesses. (Von Pohl, G., (1932). *Erdstrahlen als Krankheitserreger*. Hubertus-Verlag Diessen vor München.)

In the course of radiesthetic research, around 14 different energy systems have been demonstrated. For practical purposes, it is sufficient, in our experience, to know about the terrestrial **Diagonal Grid** (Diagonalnetzgitter - DNG), also known as the Curry Grid, as it was scientifically described for the first time by doctor Manfred Curry; and the cosmic **Global Grid** (Globalnetzgitter - GNG), also known as the Hartmann Grid, since it was scientifically described for the first time by doctor Ernst Hartmann. Both **grids** present exciting energies, similar to a **water vein** and the **Plant Growth Laser** (Pflanzenwachstumslaser - PWL) named by Oberbach, which is a stimulating bioenergetic phenomenon that manifests chiefly in damp walls in which electric lines have been installed.

In addition, a building's method of construction, electrical equipment, mirrors, metallic objects, stones, souvenirs, pictures, and many other aspects must be taken into account. Freshly renovated antique furniture can (negatively) influence the geopathic atmosphere just as much as freshly painted walls or newly bought carpets that are placed in the wrong cardinal direction. Carpets, through their symbolism, do have a direction in which they flow.

The surroundings of a house to be tested should also be considered. The more complex the geopathic atmosphere becomes, the more experience and intuition are required of the tester. A possible zero field should also be tested. Zero fields are usually not noticed by dowsers or pendulum users, since in the area of mental testing, one only finds what one is asking a question about.

When we reside in the same location for a long time, balanced room energy is most beneficial to our health and productivity. An energetic zero field (generated, for example, by a power line) or the exciting energies of a grid line or water vein weaken our own energy in a state of rest and favor degenerative processes. In humans, a PWL promotes spasms and neck tension, though in certain plants it promotes growth (for example in ferns). In places where we spend a large amount of time (like the places we sleep), all external energetic anomalies have a stimulating effect. Each person's reaction, however, is individual.

Among both plants and animals, there are fleers from radiation and seekers of radiation. Among the plants that seek radiation are elder and comfrey, plants that also help us to harmonize exciting lines and water veins for precisely this reason. As we have already alluded to, horses, dogs, and cows are fleers from radiation. Bees, ants, and cats, in contrast, are seekers of radiation.

Observation in nature teaches us many things. Trees that grow on exciting lines often have a bark structure that grows out of the ground and tends toward the left, are stunted, and have little foliage. It is consequently also important to become more familiar with natural phenomena and to observe nature in order to determine possible energetic irregularities or exciting energies, and also to become aware of corresponding sources of help.

Some experiences with stimulating energies and zero fields follow:

We were permitted to test classrooms in different school buildings. In one case, the exciting energy was so strong that three different teachers were incapable of keeping the restless pupils under control. Two of the teachers were fired. After the place was geopathically harmonized, the entire class behaved normally and the third teacher was able to remain. In other cases, we discussed the performance and behavior of individual pupils with the teachers and observed them over a long period of time with a subtle energetic focus. The fact remains that unintelligent pupils don't become intelligent and intelligent pupils don't become unintelligent because of a water vein. But the result of observing the pupils was so striking that one ought to be quite motivated to have school buildings tested. In Japan, today as in the past, hardly anyone builds a house without consulting the "energy expert." After explanations and agreement with their high school students, teachers interested in bioenergetic phenomena tested different places in the school. The result was always the same, even for pupils who didn't believe in the whole matter. Great students were, in the vibrationally very stimulating places, indeed still good, but no longer great, and some of them were also more tired and less active. Less gifted students performed better in highly harmonious places and were more active and interested.

A newly built school building in southern Germany attracted attention when instead of romping around during breaks, the pupils lay around on the floor, tired. The test revealed a complete zero field in the entire school building – brought about by a special metal girding of the building. The pupils, and naturally also the teachers, were consequently not being supplied with bioenergy during the school hours, sitting instead (and probably still sitting today) in a Faraday Cage.13 Unfortunately, the school's directors did not listen to the local naturopath and did not take any measures.

After her classroom had been freshly painted, a music school teacher noticed that her pupils were very tired. This was all the more surprising, since in the music school the pupils normally clap and jump around. In this room as well, the test revealed a lacking bioenergetic field, which meant no life *energy. After the painted walls were harmonized and an energy stone was placed, the pupils felt better again and were as active and lively as before.*

Even these few selected examples already show how great our responsibility is toward children and animals – both of which are, so to speak, at our mercy. It is high time we rediscover the ancient knowledge and, above all, apply and put it into practice: School buildings, hospitals, workplaces, animal stalls and cages should be bioenergetically tested – many physical and psychological problems in both animals and people would then be gently resolved.

It is possible with the Tensor and an appropriate systematic approach to analyze the bioenergetic atmosphere. Still, even with much practice and experience, geopathic testing is becoming more and more problematic, since it is necessary to take into consideration many influences, which contribute to our contemporary so-called quality of life, as possible interferences to our testing and interpretations. Since water is an unbelievably potent informational pool (cf. Chapter 9), swimming pools, swimming ponds, and biotopes can also become bioenergetic problems, while with the appropriate knowledge, they can possibly also become bioenergetic blessings.

We should generally regard so-called measures for disturbance suppression with skepticism. They usually do bring about an energetic improvement ranging from disturbance to a zero field; however they usually form a definitive energetic zero field, which is felt as positive at the outset with regard to the energetic disturbance, but in the long term saps one's vitality. Good radiesthetists also try to give due attention to the spiritual and subtle energetic complexity of the system that is the "living space." Not only the knowledge of a Feng Shui consultant or geomancer is helpful, but also **what is in resonance with our own knowledge and insight.**

5.3   Ley lines and vortices

Geomancy is probably the oldest interdisciplinary science in the world. It was used, on the one hand, for the people's benefit (religious and ritual sites, healing centers, and salt roads), but was also intentionally employed during war. From Alexander the Great to Adolf Hitler, many knowing or well-advised rulers carried out their campaigns on ley lines so that their armies would perform better while needing less food and sleep. All of the commanders' bunkers in the Third Reich were also said to have been located on ley line crossings. Blanche Merz mentions the Indo-Chinese traditional writings stating that the art of generals was based on geomancy. It was required of the high commander that he be experienced in atmospheric, planetary, and cosmic-terrestrial phenomena.

It is possible that the powerful of this world were always initiates who had secret knowledge, or who at least had among their advisors people who knew. As a matter of natural law, Good and Evil are always strong in equal measure. The common people were, in part, intentionally kept at a distance from geomantic knowledge.

Among many peoples, this knowledge was usually passed on only orally, and there was thus always the risk of its being lost. The subtle knowledge was, in the ancient cultures, usually only given to initiates, to chosen individuals who had corresponding specific experience and the willingness to work on this knowledge for their entire lives. This also explains why many ancient texts can be perhaps literally understood, but not understood with respect to their subtle energetic content, which cannot be comprehended without a code to decipher it. (cf. in this connection: Berner-Hürbin, A. (1997). *Hippokrates und die Heilenergie*. Schwabe Basel).

Since man has an electrically functioning nervous system and magnetic blood characteristics, he can, even if he is not sensitive enough, react to the earth's magnetism, in other words, enter into resonance, even without having knowledge. Today we are faced with the unfortunate fact that in a world where artificial radiations are ignored and not felt, bioenergetic earth radiations (even when they are of an electromagnetic nature) are of course hardly taken seriously and thus not felt or estimated to have any harmful influence.[14]

The Englishman Alfred Watkins is considered to be the one who rediscovered geomantic phenomena in the modern era. He discovered a number of churches and chapels, all of which are located on a special energetic line connecting several towns whose names end in -ley, -lay, and -leigh (from Old English and Old French, with the meaning "hidden forest path"). For this reason, lines of force are often referred to throughout the world as **ley lines**.

The straight line is evidently a geomantic feature that must have been familiar as such to ancient cultures. They can be encountered in the most diverse regions of the world. Thus we know of the so-called Nazca Line in Peru, for example, whose significance no one is really able to unravel today. In Indonesia, Buddhist temple complexes are said to be placed in such a way that they are located on a single line; in Ireland, prehistoric hill forts are connected with each other by fairy paths regarded to be straight; and in Cairo, mosques should be aligned on a straight line with respect to one another. (cf. Devereux, P., (1991). *Das Gedächtnis der Erde*, AT CH-Aarau, p.233). In this regard, Watkins quite likely discovered and described the remnants of an archaic, culturally very deeply rooted (landscape) structure.

Ley lines must be imagined as lines with a specific, particularly strong energetic radiation and a special, complex energetic structure. Ley lines are, from a quantitative and qualitative point of view, extraordinary. Like human DNA and many other archaic structures on our planet, they present a double helix structure.

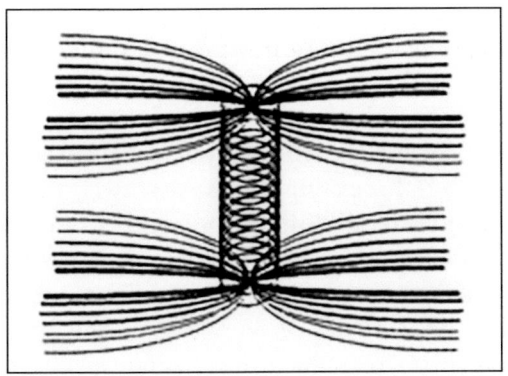

Figure 10: Double helix – double helix structure: This structure is found again and again in nature, e.g. in bioenergetically optimal water. Also, human DNA is structured as a double helix. (Illustration: BIONIK AG)

According to our testing experience, we can picture the ley line network of the earth like the human body's system of blood vessels: it provides a fundamental supply. In addition, there are the well-known large aortas, which are located on the most important points throughout the entire world, some of which have received names from geomancers, such as the Grail Line, Cosmic Line, and so on. And small and even minute vessels, analogous to the human capillary system, are also testable.

Blanche Merz, the Swiss building biologist and pioneer in the field of bioenergy, is silent on this fact, as well as on negative changes occurring in ley lines and vortices. Still, all of her books are worth reading, since she has contributed much that is essential to the perception of vortices and to making them known. Many riddles, however, remain to be solved on this subject – particularly changes in these places need to be perceived and understood. And it is becoming increasingly important to react in a healing manner to places that have become bioenergetically ill.

Ley lines and vortices can also be systematically – that is, directly and comprehensibly – tested. The complex energetic characteristics of a vortex or ley line can be made comprehensible mainly by testing polarities. Unfortunately, we were forced, with the direct testing method, to discover that many vortices and ley lines are no longer healthy, and accordingly no longer correspond to their well-known vibrational patterns.

Ley lines and vortices are, in part, massively disrupted by renovations – of churches and chapels, for example – and otherwise primarily by transmitter antennas and stations. This phenomenon seems not to have been noticed in other forms of testing. A possible explanation for this difference, which we have not yet found in the literature, could be the following: A pendulum gives a "yes" as an answer to the question, "Is this a vortex?", since a vortex remains a vortex – for positive as for negative. The question of whether it is a healthy or sick vortex is not posed. In this way, the mind-boggling figure of 15 **Bovis units** tested by experienced radiesthetists in places of power that were also experienced by ourselves as unhealthy, can be explained: The intensity as well as the degree of force remains present in an energetically sick vortex, but in an inverse form. Direct testing registers this fact, while mental testing apparently does not, since the corresponding question is not posed. In addition to this, vortices visited by crowds of tourists, for example, change during the course of the day; thus the time of day we test is also essential.

Vortices are unbelievably vital and complex configurations. Precisely due to the vivacity of their systems and interaction, geomantic phenomena are for us – at least at the present time – not definitive, and still very difficult to understand and describe. The following story, which we experienced and tested ourselves, should serve to illustrate the vitality of vortices.

Next to our house there was a large, undeveloped field on which a house was to be built. On the evening after the excavator started moving the earth, our neighbors, who are also proficient with the Tensor and bioenergetically sensitive, phoned to ask what was happening energetically, since they were feeling very unwell in their home and the Tensor indicated disturbed bioenergy. Our house, too, felt uneasy and distressed. We knew that a small ley line ran in the North-South direction straight through the freshly agitated terrain. With my neighbors as testing partners and witnesses, I came to the realization that precisely this ley line – which at the moment, for un-

derstandable reasons, was indicating disturbed bioenergy – was moving away from the construction site in the direction of our house and that of our neighbors. This ley line initially revealed itself as energetically elusive, jittery, and then the next day went straight through our house and our neighbors' (North-South axis), suffering, moaning and groaning – it was sick. I then treated this line like an ill person in a state of shock. After about three weeks, it became calm and energetically intact. We and our neighbors are gladdened by its presence... And after the changes brought about by construction, it has not returned to its former location.

> *"Intelligence is present at every point in space and can be acted upon through the power of thought."*
> Nicola Tesla, *The Wall of Light*

6. THE EARTH AS AN ORGANISM

6.1 The fundamental interconnectedness

Living, self-organizing systems have a certain autonomy with respect to their environment. This does not mean, however, they are isolated: They are in constant interaction with their environment, and this interaction determines not only the organization, network pattern, flow of energy, and cycles, but is of fundamental importance for the new scientific conception of life. We must probably take leave of a world in which space and time were held to be absolute and could be explained mechanistically. According to the view of Fritjof Capra (born 1939), two themes run like a leitmotif through all of physics, themes that are also fundamental themes of all mystical traditions: the **fundamental networkedness and mutual interdependence** of all phenomena, and the **laws of interaction,** according to which existing things are engendered out of the cosmic vacuum and are based on the transmission of information and energy. (Capra, F., (1988). *Uncommon Wisdom: Conversations with Remarkable People*, Simon & Schuster). In our scientific tradition, in contrast, the idea of **fundamental building blocks** is very strongly rooted.

Statements by scientists like Fritjof Capra and Ervin László (*Science and the Reenchantment of the Cosmos: The Rise of the Integral Vision of Reality (2006)*, Inner Traditions) help us to understand test experiences in the geomantic and geopathic domains and to better categorize and interpret them. Nature cannot be reduced to basic units, but must be totally and completely understood through its own congruity. Things exist because of their mutual connections; an organism is a totality of organs acting on one another, a purposefully subdivided Whole. This view of the universe as a networked tissue of connections is typical, for example, of the Eastern, and particularly the Buddhist body of thought. The ancient Greeks, too, had a similar conception of the universe: The earth **not only behaves like an organism, but seems to truly be an organism.**

6.2 The meaning, types, and consequences of the interaction between geopathic and geomantic phenomena

The expression geopathy is a modern term and today generally refers to the illness-provoking effect of the phenomena arising in the earth's subsurface, such as water veins and exciting terrestrial lines. γαῖα [Gaia] or γῆ [gae] stands for the earth. πάθος [pathos] is an expression that has a multitude of meanings, such as to suffer, endure, **fate, destiny**, calamity, misfortune, illness, pain, mental suffering, sorrow, passion, emotion, **event**, and occurrence. All of these meanings are, with the term geopathy, in reference to the earth.

The word geomancy is also not ancient; today the term is usually interpreted to mean "prophecy from the earth" and the teaching that is concerned with the interpretation of earth forces. The term is composed of γαῖα [Gaia] and μαντεία [manteia] = **prophecy** which, on the whole, can be extended to the meanings of gift of sight, divination, statement of an oracle, oracle site, and questioning of the oracle.

If we consider, from a linguistic point of view, the words geopathy and geomancy in their entire span of meaning in Greek, we confirm a semantic overlapping – something that for a new explanatory approach is not uninteresting. Questioning an oracle, a statement of an oracle, or a prophecy (from the earth) quite certainly has to do with fate, destiny, misfortune, pain, and passion. Translated into practical everyday life: The exciting effects of lines in the terrestrial grid system (Curry Grid) depend on the ley lines' state of health. **The geomantic state of Mother Earth determines the geopathic state.**

As we have already mentioned, it is thanks to the doctors Manfred Curry and Ernst Hartmann that the terrestrial grid and the cosmic grid (Hartmann's Global Grid) were scientifically described for the first time and recognized as being networks of energy of a specific quality (exciting energies): Silicon crystals in the earth's crust focus earth energies originating from eruptions in the earth's interior, causing them to manifest energetically on the earth's surface in regular, gridlike intervals. (Crystals "focus" energies.) Regular? Basically yes, but they are often – and more and more so – altered by technical installations, as well as being abnormal before thunderstorms, warm and cold fronts. Through solar winds and solar eruptions, the terrestrial Curry Grid lines are reflected and thrown back from the cosmos to the earth in altered cardinal directions as the cosmic Hartmann Grid.

In November 1995 in a house in Maloja, Switzerland, the Curry Grid was tested in the abnormal form of a fan. Only two years earlier, this energy grid had revealed itself in its normal, previously described net form. What had happened? Two hundred meters from the house in question, a power line (in a nature reserve, it is to be noted) had been installed, supplying not only the house with abnormal energies, but also providing the surrounding nature with an energetic zero field. Trees and plants were no longer being supplied with subtle energy; they could no longer breathe. The solution to the problem was offered by nature herself. In Maloja there are many stones. Using relational testing of the power line, stones were chosen that were placed in the form of a cross (a symbol tested with the Tensor) before the disruptive power poles in seeming wilderness (also using relational testing). Immediately after laying the stones, the Curry Grid was tested as normal and the surrounding nature could breathe again. The bioenergy began to flow once more. The residents of the house immediately experienced better health. The stone installation is checked every year following the great snowfall. With such installations, the important thing is the interaction of the force of the stones, their relationship to each other, and the symbolism.

For this reason, such "energetic installations" should be regularly checked in order to guarantee their positive effect. The experience of such an energy installation is staggering.

After the tsunami in January 2006, we tested both reversed polarities (in nature and people) and a reversed energy flow (in the ley lines). It took weeks before all of this was calm once again and directed in the former pathways.

The energy lines produced by the earth are, according to our current view, not fundamentally irritating or illness-producing; but rather they are lines that radiate a particular stimulating energy, about which it has been known for ages that they should not determine the places where we spend a great deal of time (sleeping and work places).

It is similar with water veins. Good, healthy water has no irritating energy. An energetically healthy stream or lake will always present an ordered, constructive bioenergetic vibrational field. In the border zones of water veins, as well as of streams and rivers, natural turbulences occur. These turbulences vivify the water, giving it power, so to speak, but for humans they have an exciting effect. Being exposed to the exciting effect above a water vein during the night in the resting phase is not the same as the identical exciting effect during the day by a small stream, when we experience it as stimulating refreshment.

In former times, people knew more about the different earth and water energies. They knew, for example, such locations should be avoided as resting places (not least through their observation of plants and animals), but such locations could be used for rituals and healing places. Through knowledge of the informational potential of water (cf. Chapter 8) in connection with earth and cosmic energies, in every sanctuary in ancient Greece, for example, springs were used as energy transformers. In sanctuaries all over the world we can find similar practices. The spring on Kramgasse in the city of Bern, Switzerland, presents the same system of transformation over a ley line as is demonstrated, in exemplary fashion, in the ancient Greek vortex of Delphi with at least twelve springs.

We can probably assume that on our planet, without civilizing, technical influences, there would be no disruptive energies in the sense of chaotic, disintegrating energy patterns. People in today's world – in any case, in the West – have to a large extent lost the knowledge of how to deal with specific energetic qualities. That these specific energies are becoming of decisive importance in connection with the interaction and intensification of technical pollutants, that is, they are being bioenergetically disrupted and thus capable of acting in a way that is harmful to our health, is not the fault of our Blue Planet.

In the course of our research and tests over the last few years, we saw that the ley line system and terrestrial grid system are networked. In this network, the ley line system is hierarchically higher than the grid, as we mentioned above. (We had previously tested the cosmic grid [Hartmann Grid] as being independent from the ley line system.) We have the opportunity of testing, at least partially, the networks demonstrated by recent physics and thereby being able to understand them at least approximately.

The great natural laws are being employed in the most recent developments in electronics. Most experts and users of electronics are lacking in knowledge about the deeper connections that go beyond the material level to the point of subtle energetic laws that are applied, on a coarser level, in computer science. Otherwise, a sense of awe before nature would likely be present to a greater degree, for the entire internet reflects the laws of creation. It is the image of knowledge that has always been present in the so-called information pool, since this knowledge arises from the laws of the universe. The energies in our conceivable cosmos and in creation, as far as we are able to work with them, function according to information and networking. The material level of the internet is the reflection of something much greater: the laws that are found at the basis of creation. In this vein, the tremendous developments in electronic knowledge over recent years certainly belong in this era of holistic paradigm shift.

As we realized that the ley line network is hierarchically higher than the geopathic grid, it follows that the quality of the grid systems depends on the quality of the ley line network – which does not reveal itself as a regular grid. Indeed, the exciting energy of the terrestrial Curry Line, for example, is no longer tested to be disturbed the moment the corresponding higher-level ley line is energetically satisfactory.

The same holds true for water veins. It seems that it is not yet well known in radiesthetic circles how ill a large portion of our earth's guidance system and its (likewise famous) ley lines are.

Ley lines have a predilection for hills, elevations (including church towers), and mountain peaks.

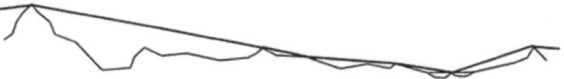

Figure 11: Terrain cross section. (Illustration: BIONIK AG)

Tragically, broadcast stations and antennas are also installed in these places, since from a technical point of view it is recognized that vibrations, tones, and so on are of greater quality in the ether when they pass between elevated locations. From a subtle energetic point of view, the reason for the improved effect is to be found in the ley line. And here also lies the drama. In Germany and other relatively flat countries, church towers are used for the installation of mobile phone antennas. Since, as it is known that churches (in any case the older ones) were built on ley lines, the repercussions resulting from the grids, which are changing in more and more serious ways and becoming "disruptive," are certainly clear to the attentive reader. In this connection, we are going to be less and less "in control," at least as long as we understand the geomantic law of resonance only on the technical level. Everything is connected with everything! We already find in the prayer of Nicholas of Flüe a geomantic process, anticipating the statements of the most modern physics.[16]

As a logical consequence of networkedness, when powerful ley lines are disrupted by human installations or by problematic weather situations, portions of grids and bodies of water are negatively affected. If the hierarchically higher ley line system is negatively influenced energetically, and as this negative influence is usually transferred – sometimes locally, sometimes more widely – to the hierarchically lower terrestrial Curry Grid (DNG), our efforts must consequently be directed, above all, to healing the "sick" ley lines; that is, we must address the cause and not the symptoms. Some experiences have shown that Curry Lines in the area of intact ley lines can indeed be found with the Tensor according to our method (they have their specific exciting characteristics) and do not present a fundamental negative test result (that is, danger) for humans.

The price we are paying in the area of our subtle energetic quality of life for technical progress is demonstrated by the fact that practically all over the world, with the Tensor, dowsing rod, or pendulum, we are testing cosmic and terrestrial grids as well as water veins as a "disturbance." If ancient peoples such as the Greeks of antiquity, the ancient Egyptians, the ancient Indians and Tibetans, and many other archaic peoples knew how to apply the specific qualities of particular terrestrial or cosmic energetic lines for healing, rituals, and many other purposes, we can assume that these energetic lines were still energetically undisturbed, highly intense, and specific.

Today's reports about military technical installations such as HAARP (Free, B. & Dr. Hynaar, (2001). *HAARP, Mindcontrol,* Pantha Reo and Amun-Verlag), and other partially secret military installations that greatly damage the ley line network – and consequently also damage grids, water, and water veins – are very alarming. As a result, a great deal has changed in the field of earth energy research in recent years, a situation that calls on us to think, test, and take personal responsibility. In this context, the classical descriptions and studies of Curry, Hartmann, Endrös, and Metzler[17] are still of fundamental importance, but now appear to be somewhat outdated.

Further bioenergetic research must be urgently directed to finding and demonstrating ways for vortices and ley lines to be energetically stabilized.

In addition to concrete measures it is, not the least, a matter of importance to once again recognize and experience the power of thought. In the domain of subtle energies above all, it is useful to employ our thoughts consciously and intentionally, to learn how to enter a vortex with mental discipline, and to be ready to give new impulses to weakened energy points through rituals with like-minded people (a group is always stronger than an individual person). In this age of electrosmog, it is often necessary for such places to be energetically cared for on a regular basis. **It will no longer be possible to heal human beings without previously healing the entire landscape (and thus the earth).**

In this connection, we must mention Marko Pogačnik (born 1944), a trained sculptor who seeks to link art with everyday life and agriculture. He places specially sculpted stones in particular places and through this helps the organism that is the earth with a kind of earth acupuncture. His work is now endorsed and supported by a group of people throughout Europe. Pogačnik gives lectures all over Europe, is the author of several valuable books (on geomancy, feeling and healing the earth, and elemental beings), and is director of the Hagia Chora School of Geomancy in Munich.[18]

We will also be involved in more landscape-rehabilitating projects in the future. Ley lines, as well as streams, rivers, and lakes, can be optimized with bioenergetic knowledge. The development of simple, affordable measures against the disruptions caused by transmitters and antennas is of increasing importance, as the latter naturally cannot be harmonized by the power of thought alone.

In the context of a seminar, it was proven that with bioenergetic knowledge and mental work and without any technical aids, a healthy vortex can be created out of an energetically disturbed one. The place that was treated was tested by all the participants before and after the course. Not only the test results were identical, but subjective perceptions were as well – such as perceiving a different scent, the beech leaves shining as they had not been before, and so on. The fact that a pair of ducks took a siesta during the "action" in the middle of the seminar participants does not prove anything, it is true, but it does speak for harmonizing energies. Such a place would need to be energetically cared for in the meanwhile to have a chance to be stabilized in the new, optimized energy.

In this connection, intensive observation and perception of nature is important, even to the extent – for those who are able – of communicating with the elemental beings. An example of a plant that reveals a very strong, specific radiation is the mistletoe, a plant that already occupied a special position among the Celtic Druids. Someone who observes nature with a subtle energetically trained eye will learn to understand much about networkedness and about the geopathic and geomantic situation, as well as the technical influences on the latter.

Nature offers us a great many aids and healing resources – as well as aids and healing resources for sick nature herself. It is up to us to find them. We are faced with the challenge to discover new things in today's era of omnipresent, rapid upheaval. It is not sufficient to continue working with only the ancient knowledge of plants and other domains. During the times of Paracelsus (1493-1541), Samuel Hahnemann (1755-1843), the herbal priest Künzle (1857-1945), or Dr. Edward Bach (1868-1936), today's disruptive environmental conditions did not yet exist. Both nature and the human body were differently informed and reacted differently accordingly. The investigation of ancient subtle energetic knowledge should form the solid foundation for contemporary subtle energetic innovation, which includes people, animals, and plants, with the goal of harmonizing and healing in an environment that is, one must admit, rather threatening.

6.3 Geopathy and geomancy as consciously experienced resonance

The more consciously, sensitively, and conscientiously we seek to experience and understand geopathic and geomantic phenomena, the more our own non-illumined parts of ourselves radiate, become visible, and are able to be experienced and suffered. We become a mirror of ourselves: consciously entering into resonance, experiencing what happens during resonance in silence, and feeling and experiencing how geopathic and geomantic phenomena release and dissolve old patterns, images, and sentiments, as is familiar in meditation. In this way, physical, mental, and spiritual processes can be initiated. Therefore it is also necessary to accept possible physical pain and mental and spiritual difficulties as expressions of transformation. Each person has the opportunity to become a well-tuned instrument. It is advisable, however, not to expose ourselves to these untrained sensations that arise from the experience of resonance alone. With another person or a like-minded group, we generally feel more at ease and also have witnesses for ostensibly "inexplicable" energetic events.

Today each person has the possibility of accessing subtle energetic knowledge and of experiencing resonance with geopathic and geomantic phenomena. Through the process that can be initiated here (searching for your **own** place of power), each person also has the opportunity to arrive at his own energetic home, his own subtle center, provided that he directs his consciousness, in silence, toward the laws of this knowledge: toward **resonance**. Then he may also discover that he can enter into resonance with his birthplace, with the place he currently lives, or with a far-away place he feels drawn to and visits. We can also begin to understand this resonance as a kind of affectionate turning toward particular places.

Through the law of resonance, geopathic and geomantic phenomena show themselves to be something like an exchange between matter and spirit – between body, soul, and spirit – which, with some practice, should also be able to be experienced as such. By consciously experiencing the earth's forces and the energetic lines, we enter more optimally into resonance with the forces of nature, thanks to which we can better integrate ourselves into nature and her laws. This inspires the soul and gives clarity to the spirit. Perhaps this conjecture points us toward the path to a better and truer life – to a place where we feel embedded in the wholeness of the universe and can define ourselves within this wholeness.

"Research is seeing what others don't see and thinking what others haven't thought."
Nobel prizewinner Hans-Adolf Krebs

7. THE UNDERSTANDING OF LIFE – RESONANCE, INFORMATION, COMMUNICATION

The understanding of life presupposes knowledge of the interactions that take place in the extremely complex and dynamic organization of living systems, with a broad scope, and not just exploring the structure of dead organisms. Life and its history can thus be the object of research only of disciplines and scientists that think in a system that functions as a whole, without losing view of this whole.

Life can be described not only in quantitative and mechanical terms such as force, matter, and energy, since **life, in its essential characteristics, is metaphysical, metachemical, metamaterial, metaenergetic, and metamechanical.**

Science has driven out the gods and fairies. Material world affairs can – as people believe today – be understood without them. But can we truly grasp the abstract truth of life with the means currently at our disposal? Can man extend his gaze down to the utmost foundations of the world? Some scientists may actually believe that they will soon have God's plan in their hands. But the question of whether living beings can ever know absolute truth, the utmost foundation of reality, implies the question of whether living beings are at all capable of understanding themselves, or life, at an absolute level. Every living being is itself a part of this holistic reality.

If we recognize physics as the highest authority for describing reality, the question suggests itself: What kind of truth does physics describe, after all? Or should we turn instead to theology in order to better understand life? For **re-ligio** (Lat. religere = reconnect) is related to resonance. True religion is to be found in the place where there is resonance, where one feels secure, that is, reconnected. Re-ligio has very much to do with true life, and true life is life lived in resonance in compliance to the laws.

According to Aristotle, the shape of living beings is brought about by means of a particular, form-giving force. This force that moves and gives form was for him the soul, which he also designated as entelechy. In his view, the body is οργανον [organon], or the instrument of the soul. Paracelsus spoke of the spiritual body, the "archeus," as the form-giving authority that creates the body. He understood archeus as a spiritual principle, a creative, ordering intelligence. The astronomer Johannes Kepler (1571-1630), in his work *Harmonices Mundi* (1619), also examined the phenomena of forces in a particular manner, asking himself the question of what is actually at work behind what we see. This question moved him deeply and he came to the following conclusion: **The cause of form is not to be found in matter, but in activity. The real world exists only in the mathematical harmony inherent in things. The ever-changing qualities of the things we can perceive with our senses represent a lower plane of reality and do not possess veritable being.**

From these statements of prominent thinkers, it follows that not adaptation, for example, but rather creation and cooperation, communication and information, **subtle energetic forces** may be the formative forces that are active at the basis of life and evolution. When we examine the reports from current biophoton research, we learn that cancer cells, for example, do not communicate with their environment, communication being normal for healthy cells. In this connection, the question arises of whether illness is not the consequence of an (intercellular) disruption of communication. And when we raise the question of life, the question of death naturally also arises – that is, the **dissolution of structures and information.**

In order to explain the continual, if by no means uniform or linear, evolution of existing things, we must add an element of interaction that is not **only** bioenergy. More and more scientists recognize how important this element is: **the element of information**. Information as a real and operative factor that influences evolutionary processes in all areas and parts of the known universe. The Russian researcher Vladimir I. Vernadsky (1863-1945) had already prophesied that future scientists would extend the notion of life to include additional factors besides matter and energy, and that one of these would have to be the factor of information. (Vernadsky, V.I., (1967). *The Biosphere* (Russian). Moscow.)

In-formare means to give form from within. Thus bioenergy, by means of information, becomes **directed** energy (cf. entelechy). Information seems to be a subtle, almost momentary, non-transient connection between things in different places in space at different points in time. As for its temporal existence, it is regarded as a form of memory in both nature and in interpersonal and transpersonal communication: Information is the supertemporal reaction of the entity characterized as a quantum vacuum to things and events in space and time. All things and events that take place in space and time leave behind traces in this vacuum. They inform it, and the informed vacuum has an effect, in its turn, on things and events: At the very basis of life, the fundamental law of giving and receiving, of sowing and reaping is at work.

Much may still be unknown about the structure of the vacuum, but today it is at least clear that it engenders coherence between the particles that are embedded in it. This coherence-engendering characteristic of the vacuum is not only explainable in the sense of an energy transfer; it is rather the transfer of a particular form of information: physically operative, active information or in-formation. It is thus fully possible today to assume that the quantum vacuum is not only a sea of energy, but also an ocean of information.

Vernadsky alluded to the significance of information as an additional factor besides matter and energy. Alexander S. Presman, as early as the 1960s, also held the conviction that the informative aspect of electromagnetic fields is more significant than the magnetic and energetic aspect. (Presman, A.S. (1968). *Electromagnetic fields and life*. Moscow).

A new view of the universe based on the rediscovery of the Akashic field, the field residing in the vacuum known as the holistic field, is being studied by the physicists of the 21st century. In this view, the universe is a highly integrated, coherent system. An essential characteristic is information, which is produced, preserved, and conveyed by and between all parts. This characteristic is fundamental; it transforms a universe that is groping from one form of evolution to the next into a powerfully networked system that builds upon the defining information that it has already produced.

A cosmic field that lies at the basis of everything in the world and that connects everything corresponds to an apparently immortal intimation that has always appeared in traditional forms of cosmology and metaphysics. In antique civilizations, it was known that space is not empty, but rather represents the origin and memory of all things that exist and that have ever existed. In this sense, the prophecy that in the Age of Aquarius, ancient knowledge would be newly discovered is being fulfilled for science as well. It has been said that the internet is actually a modern expression of ancient cosmological knowledge, an expression – albeit on the lowest, most material level – of fundamental notions and laws.

Information is neither energy nor matter. It is a third entity, which can be compared to a message from a sending to a receiving system. The signals transmitted can be letters, characters, symbols, or numbers. In the realm of bioinformation, they are electromagnetic frequency patterns. Information must be appropriate to the system, in other words, it must enter into resonance with the receiver. As we have seen, Popp proves that transmission of information in living systems takes place by means of ultraweak signals. Accordingly, biological information is only active when it is so weak that it falls under so-called broadband noise.

The thought that there may be direct physical effects of thoughts, imagination, and feelings on the material world, that our thoughts and feelings are no longer inseparable from those of other people, that what is deepest within us may be exposed and unprotected from the outside, and similar notions, run contrary to many of the basic tenets and the basic disposition of our European culture and Western civilization, not in the least as a result, most likely, of the high value accorded to individuality, autonomy, and freedom, which have been cultivated and developed in the West for years. This thought, however, also opens up unimagined collective possibilities on the one hand (like group visits to places of power), and on the other hand, explains many ailments and illnesses that are often the consequence of violating cosmic laws.

The greater one's consciousness and knowledge about these interactions and the greater one's understanding of life, the more effective one's own protection and the more efficient one's own activity will be. Man has the free will to choose in which resonance he wishes to place himself, and from this follows the people with whom he will communicate. But information only flows when the sender and receiver are attuned and genuine. This is applicable on both small and large scales, on both the cellular level and human life. We are thus not unprotected and at the mercy of anything when we take our place in the Whole and understand its laws.

Both laboratory experiments and anthropologists' observations testify to the reality of a transpersonal connection between individuals, but this is not everything: Archaeology and history reveal that such connections have also been present, and most likely continue to be present, between entire peoples and cultures (for example, the simultaneous construction of pyramids in Egypt and Peru). Subconscious, spontaneous contacts between cultures seem to have been a widespread phenomenon, as we can see in the works of art of different civilizations. Annie Berner-Hürbin explains transcultural parallels only partially in terms of contacts between the peoples. She also understands these phenomena as largely a matter of morphic resonance.

It seems that the self-organization of life takes place essentially by means of informational exchange and communication (when resonance is present). **The carrier of information is what we understand by the concept**

of bioenergy. This is what differentiates living systems categorically from dead ones and what makes them living beings. Life is both a natural and an ideational phenomenon. **The interface between spirit and matter could truly be information.** If we were to suppose that geomancy is categorized, according to our current understanding, in the (energetic) interface between matter and spirit, we must consider, as a consequence, that geomancy is information. This means that all the myths about ancient oracle sites would immediately manifest into something almost physically tangible: If we were to compare the semantic content of the word "geomancy" with the supposition that geomancy could approximately correspond to what modern physics calls information, we would come a bit closer still to the lost ancient knowledge, bridging the gap between our ostensibly different subjects.

Life is not something devoid of spirit. On the contrary, life is inspired. The Latin verb "inspirare" means "to breathe in." Man ate from the tree of knowledge and became aware of himself. This raised him, as a responsible spiritual being, above the animal world, which although it possesses a soul, is not inspired, not spiritual. Through an all-encompassing system of communication, knowledge became insight, cognition, perception of the world. Also the insight that emptiness is the creative form: All things are generated from the void, and our bodies receive their life from the middle of the void. It can thus be surmised that the vacuum is not only a sea of energy and a pool of information, but also a pool of consciousness. In this way, the world memory – formulated by mystics of all times – would be furnished with a theory.

Information is only possible when there are two partners (atoms, molecules, organs, organisms, etc.) which enter into relationship and receive and understand messages. Good information and good communication are present only when the partners are in resonance with each other.

In Delphi, one of the most important sanctuaries of ancient Greece, altered states of consciousness were used for prophecies: The seer Pythia was able to give prophecies because she was in resonance with the healing water of the Castalian Spring and the place of power where she presided as oracle, seated over the flowing water on a tripod of bronze. Her prophecies were only comprehensible, however, to those who were themselves also in energetic resonance with the seer and the place.

Here we would like to make a brief digression about our four-legged friends. Monty Roberts is world-renowned as a "horse whisperer," not least through the film of the same name. The fact is, however, that Monty Roberts is wrongly understood by most people – he doesn't whisper, but rather listens to the horses. Monty Roberts learned from nature how horses communicate with each other, for example, the mare with her foal. If this form of communication with horses, as described by Monty Roberts, is used with horses, many problems can be solved – not magically, as many think, but with Equus, the language of horses. Precisely because the sender and receiver are then in resonance – from this moment at the latest – the riding crop becomes superfluous! The same system would be imaginable for all animals, according to their species. (Roberts, M., (2002). *Die Sprache der Tiere*. Gustav Lübbe Bergisch-Gladbach.)

Information that is bound to dissipative organisms has the tendency to spread out. We can thus conclude from the most recent developments in physics that there is no life without communication, and that information is a decisive factor in the functional process of life. Different forms of therapy are based on this knowledge and work with it. Life can thus be optimized through resonant communication. If our life energy comes into being through our metabolism, then the stronger our cell communication is, the stronger our metabolism will be. Thus healing of the human body is possible, for example, through optimizing cell communication (emission of biophotons), which represents healing at a foundational level. Water presents itself as one of the most effective possibilities in this connection. Since man consists largely of water, his body can be brought into resonance, into vibrations promoting healing, by means of individually informed water. We will speak more about this in the following chapter.

Communication is thus understood as an exchange of information: Life means participating together in form-giving forces and communicating in resonance. Life is information connected with communication. What can be tested with the tensor is the sum of this – **the bioenergy**. When it is harmonious, this means that **the information and communication of the cells of the organs in the human body are functioning properly**. When the resonance is not attuned, or when almost no intercellular communication is taking place, we can, if necessary, restore the communication, the resonance between the elements in question, by using subtle energetic methods. The exact thing happens on the intercellular level in relationships between human beings. Thus we can understand the reason for therapeutic failure in certain cases: Someone (usually unconsciously) refuses to communicate, someone does not want to be open to resonance – and all of this (albeit not only) on the intercellular level.

It is well known that butterflies find their mates at a great spatial distance. Here so-called pheromones are apparently at work. The quantity of substance released into the air is, however, not enough to corroborate this explanation scientifically. Do electromagnetic fields as carriers of energy enter the picture here?

According to current understanding, such phenomena are to be explained by morphogenetic fields. We have also experienced that we learn more easily when several people are learning at the same time, since the informational fields thus created benefit each participant. Morphic fields are independent of spatial location. If we assume that morphic fields exist as a memory of the universe, without needing human participation, we ask ourselves which is more fundamental: information or resonance? In any case, certain fundamentals of **what constitutes life**, regarding the notions of **information, communication**, and **resonance**, can be defined and explained. The consequences and possibilities of these experimental results and insights – in combination with what has been learned intellectually – will now be developed with a view to their significance for therapeutic measures.

"Soul of man, how art thou like water!"
Johann Wolfgang von Goethe,
Song of the Spirits over the Waters

8. WATER – THE ENERGETIC PROPERTIES OF THE MOST IMPORTANT ELEMENT OF LIFE

8.1 Water is life

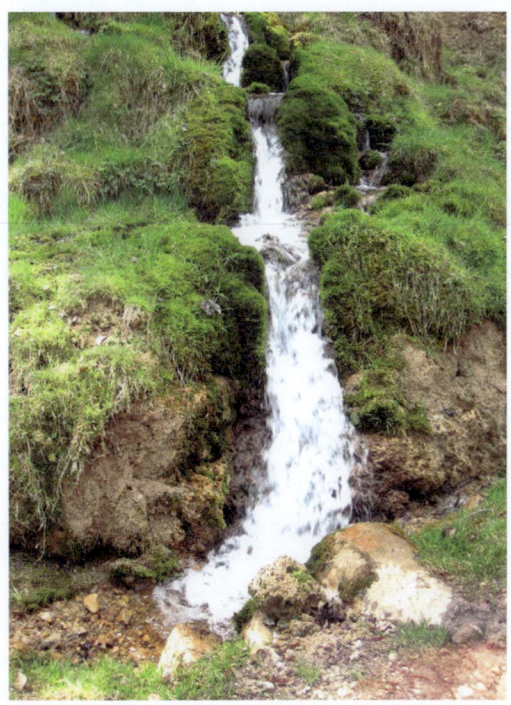

Figure 12: Spring – Sagenweid spring. (Photo: Andrea Vock)

June 1981. At the railing of a small ship in the middle of the Aegean Islands, beer cans, cola bottles, and sandwich bags are thrown into the sea. An elderly Greek woman clothed in black is smiling with wisdom and friendliness, while a little girl with chewing gum in her hand looks around, searching in vain for a trash can.

Water was sacred to ancient cultures. For millennia, special wells and springs have been venerated as holy and/or healing. For understandable reasons, water was considered in most religions and myths to be the source of life. Water is life. Survival.

It is hardly by chance that we can observe the duality present in water symbolism in all cultures. It is true that water is the source of life, but it is also the annihilator of life. Water stands for fertilization and death, for becoming and passing away. There is water from heaven and water from the depths. This apparent contradiction is due to the element's wholeness. **Water is the element in and through which information, communication, and resonance work together optimally, making life possible.**

For humans, too, the decisive nascency and development phase takes place in an aqueous solution. As the medium of the – virtual – bath, baptism and rebirth or renewal, we encounter water in the most diverse representations of ancient cultures.

It is well known that three quarters of the globe is covered by water. Around three quarters of every human, animal, and plant body is water based. Water is the only liquid that can form oceans. No substance on earth is capable of replacing water.

Water is, along with fire, air, and earth, one of the fundamental elements, suggesting that there is an archaic knowledge of ancient peoples unknown to us, a knowledge that leads further than our current understanding that raises questions about water only with regard to its chemical and physical "irregularity." For science, the "source of life" still contains many unsolved mysteries.

Our civilized society has managed to treat water with so little understanding and respect that it is a stroke of luck nowadays to find a spring in nature with truly (and energetically) good water quality. Research shows the degree to which human health depends on the quality of drinking water. It is proven that certain high quality water really has a special effect: concrete becomes harder, plants thrive better, pipelines are decalcified, and in humans, drinking specific water can normalize blood values, excrete more toxins, and strengthen the immune system. All processes of life are directly or indirectly connected to water. For this reason, water also occupies an important position in problems related to the environment.

It is increasingly urgent to rediscover and apply ancient knowledge to the subject of water. **A new consciousness in relation to water is imperative. Is our consciousness not, perhaps, our organ of resonance? This would mean that only through a NEW consciousness can we enter into the necessary resonance with water.**

8.2 The repository of vibrations: material and energetic particularities of water

A water molecule consists of two atoms of hydrogen and one atom of oxygen, which form an angle of over 100 degrees with one another. The atomic bonds are not fully absorbed for the inner bond. Thus the water molecule is outwardly active as a v-shaped dipole. The chain linkage, through hydrogen bridges to so-called clusters that results from this, is the cause of a number of water's special characteristics. Examining these in detail is beyond the scope of this book. One of the many characteristics of this life-enabling and life-sustaining liquid unexpected by chemists is the fact that water's melting and boiling points are much higher than with similar chemical compounds. We could say that water, in a certain sense, evades scientific method.

According to De Broglie's atomic model, every atom, molecule, and system has its own typical wave field. Naturally good water has, up to a specific molecular range, namely 0.695 liters (this boundary region being familiar to us with our 0.7 liter bottles, which are not nearly as fragile as larger bottles and which also permit wine to develop optimally), a spherical emanation whose outer limit is 90 cm (determined in the research carried out by the Forschungskreis e.V. für Geo-Hydro-Biologie in Igelsbach, Germany, until 1979). The signal boundary of fluoridated drinking water, in contrast, is further outside and no longer corresponds to healthy drinking water as tested according to bioenergetic norms.

Because the water molecule consists of two H atoms and one O atom, within the area of 90 cm, further concentric circles can be tested at 50 cm and 25 cm, respectively. The concrete chemical formula of water, H_2O, thus also finds expression in these subtle energetic test indications. A quantity of water over 10 liters, and accordingly the human body (approximately) as well, forms a further energy shell at 9.60 m – in a healthy, biologically intact state.

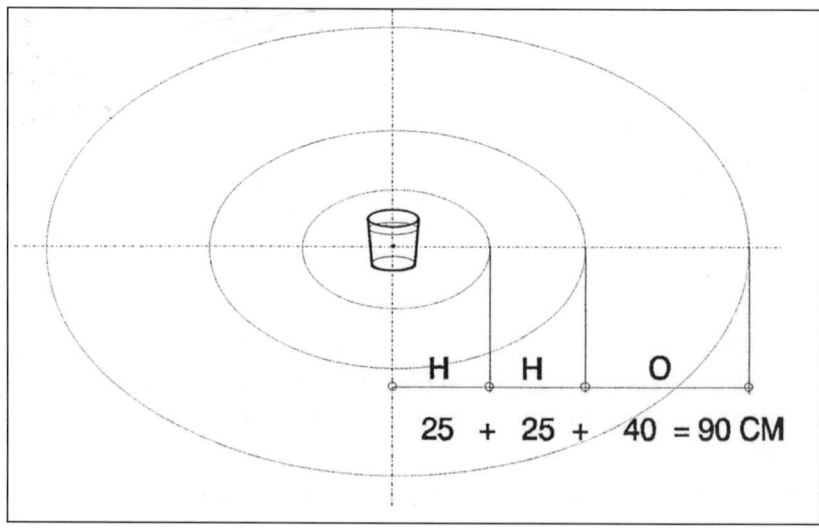

Figure 13: Sketch H2O – with ideally 0.7 liters water, the two H atoms and the O atom are bioenergetically testable in concentric circles at 25 cm and 50 cm within the 90 cm area. (Illustration: BIONIK AG)

Good water that is beneficial to all forms of life is materially and biologically pure, as well as chemically close to neutral. In addition, water has nonmaterial qualities that play an important role, still rarely taken into account today, for the health and bioenergetic state of living beings. According to our view, distilled water has, at best, short-term therapeutic value.

One of the most important characteristics of water is the fact that it can be informed. Because of this, there are still untapped possibilities waiting to be explored, both generally for health and specifically for therapy, since the bodies of humans, animals, and plants consist, after all, largely of water. Between two thirds and three quarters of the human body consists of water, and individual parts such as the interior of the cell, the blood, brain, and spinal fluid are over 90% water. Through resonant healing information, cell bonds in all dissipative organisms can be brought into healthy, harmonious vibrations, thus initiating a process of recovery in sick organisms. Bioenergetically ill lakes, rivers, and streams can also be informed in this way, a fact that can lead to the recovery of entire landscapes.

It thus appears that water possesses a kind of memory, something that certain researchers have meanwhile investigated and described.[21] Previous influences and information are stored in good water for a surprisingly long time. This can be seen as the basis for the fact that water as high potency can continue to preserve the vibrations of an active substance even when the molecules themselves have long since been diluted out of it. Thus it is possible in the human body through its water-containing parts to subtle energetically detect information from pathological vibrations originating from past serious illnesses or information from medications taken over long periods. By neutralizing these vibrations stored in the body's water, it is possible to contribute to the well-being and more stable health of the body in question.

The healing effect of homeopathy is recognized and valued in many circles today, but it continues to be attacked and branded as implausible by certain parties. Someone who only works with coarse vibrations will never understand the active principle of homeopathy. Homeopathic effects cannot be understood through classical scientific experiments and measurements. Its foundations are completely out of place in the realm of conventional biochemistry and pharmacology, belonging instead to the area of quantum phase transitions. Homeopathy is for the most part comprehensible in the context of informational and energetic medicine.

Someone who has an understanding for subtle energetic phenomena, in contrast, knows that high-potentiated dilutions of a substance have a particularly strong action. Officially, this fact is ignored in water, and purportedly harmless small quantities of toxins are deemed acceptable. This lack of understanding could lead to dramatic consequences. In the groundwater and in our swimming pools, this fact is already having a disastrous effect. Perhaps the snake of chemistry will bite its own tail when, in the future, women won't need to take hormones during menopause – it will be enough to send them to a public swimming pool. This is not a sarcastic remark, but a realization that emerges from subtle energetic, informative medicine.

Everyone treated with hormones (birth control pills, hormones for menopause, etc.) secretes through their body, their skin and pores at least the corresponding information into water. Research reports are already circulating about changes taking place in male creatures in the medium of water. Possibilities exist, however, to neutralize harmful, unhealthy information in water. Unfortunately it is very rare for authorities to concern themselves with this subtle energetic problem area of water, swimming pools, and other bathing facilities.

Fortunately the water in this country is chemically satisfactory. Indeed, water containing toxins is chemically treated to the extent that it is safe, at a coarse material level, as drinking water. At the informative level, however, water retains certain signals (for example from lead, cadmium, and nitrates) which, according to their wavelength, can be harmful to health. Our drinking water may, despite its treatment and adherence to threshold values, thus contain a significant percentage of stored information that is injurious to health. This information can be tested in the water molecules.

Naturally, water also stores beneficial information. Water from glaciers, for example, containing information from vibrations (also atmospheric) thousands of years old, has shown itself to be particularly healing. Each of the so-called healing waters also has its own typical subtle healing qualities, since it is positively informed by an energetically valuable location.

Water can also be informed or energized by symbols and forms: We may cite as an example the baptismal font of the town church in Aarau, Switzerland, presented in the form of an octahedron. The geometrical form of the octahedron intensifies subtle energy to a much greater degree than the circular form of the conventional baptismal font.

On the subject of water's mode of action and man's bioenergetic perception:

The water in the Saanen swimming pool is harmonized and energized with our bioenergetic device. The swimming athletes don't know anything about this, but they were asked to give their impressions at the end of their first day of training. The water was described as being so "silky" and "creamy," and it allowed them to move forward much more easily (a feature related to the lower surface tension due to the harmonization). Astonishingly, they recorded their best performances at the beginning of the new season.

Water study in Catalonia, Spain:

After the harmonization of an ocean bay in Spanish Catalonia, several people who knew nothing about the previous energetic treatment of the bay reported that this was now the only place where they went swimming, since nowhere else did the water feel so "silky." (Applications repeated every year since 2003.)

Due to its strongly polar molecules, water occupies a special position not only as a repository of vibrations, but also as a transmitter of vibrations.

An interaction also takes place through energy fields outside the body. Water thus has an effect on living beings without being brought into the body, and as a result – as we will discuss later – acquires a new, therapeutically interesting aspect. Let us only imagine for a moment how good we feel near a waterfall or the invigorating effect of a rushing mountain stream.

Experiment with Norbert Seiler on June 26, 1997:

In Kriens, Switzerland, on a school ground with a spring, the ideal standing location is tested for a person whose current bioenergy is shown to be in the normal range. Now the person swallows a few mouthfuls of special, energized water. The testers present notice a striking energy increase in the test person, and after a short time, a rise in energy is indicated in each control person present. The energy of the water in the spring also becomes stronger, and finally this extends, by impulses, to the entire surrounding landscape.

Such experiments have been made with different variants and in different locations. They show that the water in the human body – for better as well as for worse – informs its surroundings and is itself informed as well. (The studies of Masaru Emoto are particularly important for us in this connection.) Here the permeability of living systems is especially apparent. Water acts in every case as a transformer, not only in connection with ley lines and water (though here it does so particularly strongly). Springs generally further transmit vibrations in a more intensified state (here again, for better or worse). This knowledge was used earlier in the sacred domain, in the construction of cities (cf. the Kramgasse in the city of Bern, Switzerland), and in medicine.

8.3 Vibrational qualities of water

The nonmaterial qualities of water, its vibrational states, encompass subtle energy as a wave field and the bioinformation as modulations of energy waves, in summary: **bioenergy**. This quality is dependent on pollution and its potentialization, as well as the vibrational influence from the outside. The vibrational qualities are changed by natural (for example, meteorological) influences, features of the landscape like grottos and caves, or technical installations (transmitter stations and antennas).

By means of special spectral analysis; pictographic methods like the color plate; Kirlian photography and its successors (crystallization and drop pictures); energy potential analysis according to the method of P.M. Pfeiffer; crystallization photography according to the method of Masaru Emoto from Japan; and naturally also radiesthetically with the Tensor, the vibrational quality of water can be measured, made visible, and – with a certain amount of knowledge – analyzed. It can also be physically experienced through the kinesiological muscle test.

Following many years of activity as one of the directors of Johann Tikale's research group for geohydrobiology in Igelsbach, Germany, Norbert Seiler developed a clear, reliable system for providing reproducible indications about the energetic state of water using the BIONIK Tensor. Water can present the following vibrational qualities:

- disharmonious to the point of disruptive
- harmonious to neutral
- generally energizing
- specifically stimulating
- unipolar

Good, harmonious, energizing water must display right-polarity with the BIONIK Tensor. Left-polarity, or alternating polarities, suggests a disharmonious vibrational field. The characteristic of truly healing water is **unipolarity**, in which left- and right-polarity cancel each other out.

Water can also be dead, lifeless, and without energy. Water can be lacking in a bioenergetic field, something that occurs, for example, underneath or at a particular angle to a power line (during a 2009 seminar, this was experienced and tested with a group at the Reussspitz, in the canton of

Aargau, Switzerland). What bioenergetically lifeless water, or water whose bioenergetic structures have been destroyed, means for the Blue Planet, for humans, animals, and plants, is something we can only begin to imagine with trepidation.

Too little is spoken about the energetic pollution of water. A stream continuously regenerates itself when it is able to flow, constantly energizing itself by meandering in its natural stream bed. Turbulences vivify and purify streams and rivers and transmit new impulses and information. When a flowing body of water is corrected, the water loses its original bioenergy in the artificially determined course. It cannot renew itself and is unable to rid itself of negative information. Even without the hypothetical scenario of water pollution having taken place, because its course is being unnaturally forced, the water is energetically dead.

This is also the case for tap water. Drinking water is, in our latitudes, chemically pure and hygienically safe, it is true. But the drinking water is "pent up" in the pipes, stressed as a consequence and lifeless accordingly. The biophotons lose their radiation and, as a result, their capability of communication and resonance. We are not dying of thirst with our drinking water, but we are no longer able to provide ourselves with the refreshing vitality of the energetic, high-quality liquid – like that found around primary rocks – that would supply and vitalize our body in a bioenergetically optimal way. The water problem is similar to the subject of food and nutrition, which was described by Fritz-Albert Popp in connection with the light intensifier.

8.4 Perspective

Verifying, improving, and using appropriate water qualities is one of our goals. The practices of influencing water include harmonizing it, energizing it, and possibly storing selected information. As we have seen, because of its chemical structure, water lends itself to being informed easily, and it is extremely communicative. Thus not only water-containing organisms can be influenced through water, but geopathic and geomantic phenomena can also be changed. Conversely, water can also be influenced by geopathic and geomantic phenomena. All of this takes place within the lawful order at the foundation of the cosmos, the lawful order which is present in the connection between resonance, information, and communication.

It is instructive to test the bottled water that is available for purchase. All of the measures that are promoted as improving quality can then be tested in a personally responsible way. In addition, not every type of bioenergetically intact water is good for every organism. Whoever can help himself and, by means of relational tests, find the water that is most appropriate for himself, is fortunate. It is usually optimal to alternate between different types of good water. A practiced tester is capable of differentiating between normal, poor, and healing water, and of selecting the appropriate water for himself. The individually required quantity is also testable, something that can be important with today's tendency to make globalized statements. **The body should receive the water beneficial to it in the individually correct quantity.** Too much (which overtaxes the kidneys) is as harmful as too little.

Through our method of water therapy (cf. 9.4.2.), we were able to establish that especially the human (and animal) psyche is positively influenced, precisely because bioenergy is to be found at the juncture between body and soul, and because genuine and individually appropriate healing waters communicate intensely and inform and are highly open to resonance. In this connection we may also refer to the statement made by psychiatrist Jakob Bösch during a lecture in Solothurn, namely that the personality is reflected in water. Not only the personality, but the state of the soul is expressed in water. **Each person is his own mirror. This means that looking in the mirror in the morning can be a therapeutic approach. And it means that water, too, acts at the juncture between body and soul.** This fundamental realization is familiar to us from Grimm's fairy tales. It should continue to point the way for bioenergetic water research and water applications.

Was water then, in earlier times, man's most basic remedy of all? This question has been accompanying us for a good part of our path. If information, communication, and resonance are what define life, where should we look for healing, if not in the medium that unites these three aspects in the most optimal way?

We recently tested water and water veins along a strong, healthy ley line. All of the water presented unipolarity, a fact that would support our thesis that the majority of the earth's freshwater originally had healing properties – during a time, of course, when all the ley lines were energetically healthy.

For the present, however, it is quite interesting that water, as the well-known element in which all earthly life came to be, can fulfill the conditions that make optimal life and optimal healing possible, according to the most ancient knowledge and the most recent physics. If it is written in Genesis 1:2 (King James Version), "…and the Spirit of God moved upon the face of the waters," could this mean that at the time when the earth's organism was at its beginnings and still healthy, all water had the quality of healing, that all water was informed by the Spirit of God, that is, by a higher vibrational frequency?

For science, water still holds many unsolved mysteries. Perhaps it is good and rightly so, that the primordial soup, **the source of life**, remains a final secret. Recent research, however, shows the degree to which human health depends on the quality of drinking water. All processes of life are directly or indirectly connected with water. For this reason, water occupies an important position not only in problems related to the environment, but also in everyday life and in medicine and healing.

At the material level, water appears to be the most suitable medium for giving the body a healing impulse (water to water). The body can react to this since it contains much water itself. A part of the body's water registers signals extremely rapidly and distributes them in the body just as rapidly. In the process, the feedback in control systems is intensified to such an extent that processes gone awry are able to return to the norm.

Generally speaking, our health will develop in parallel to the qualitative development of our drinking water, and not only for hygienic reasons. For this reason it can only be recommended that we look, early enough, for affordable, truly useful measures for improving the energetic quality of our water. An effective key to health is to be found here. In this connection, each person can test, feel, and discover on his own which of the many available water improvement systems he resonates with, and not least, which system his wallet resonates with. Let us not be overly optimistic: The way world events are unfolding, no one is going to be looking after our personal well-being, specifically, our own energetically positive drinking water. There are already movements underway to privatize water. Then prices and logistics could also be manipulated by the water lobby. Here as well, more personal responsibility and knowledge are necessary.

> *"In purity and according to divine law will I carry out my life and my art."*
> Verse 5 of the Hippocratic Oath[22]

9. BIOENERGY IN HEALING

9.1 Ancient roots, ancient knowledge

Ancient peoples experienced the cosmos as a multilayered energy field with which man, with his own energy field, is constantly connected. The healers of China and India, as well as the ancient Greek doctors, understood healing processes at the level of subtle energetic phenomena. Among the shamanic peoples, too, healing was predominantly connected with the use of intuitive, clairvoyant, and spiritual forces. Energy as a physical entity was not known. In this sense, the healing methods of ancient cultures and advanced civilizations were comparable to one another. In principle, practitioners sought to heal the body through the soul.

Generally speaking, in our latitudes today, it seems that we know and value the Asian more than the European healing methods. The philosophical system of Traditional Chinese Medicine includes the concept of life energy, known as qi or chi. This energy is, under a different name, connected with teachings of the elements in India and ancient Greece. They all believed that life is composed of the different elements of nature, and that illness represents the predominance of one of these elements. It is not our purpose here, however, to analyze this force against the backdrop of the ying-yang teaching, but to ascertain that the subtle life energy we refer to as **bioenergy** has always, in a particular form, been a subject in healing and medicine and has been used knowingly for the purpose of healing. The emergence and the tradition of European medicine are fascinating and – if we look behind the scenes – they display many parallels with the Asian therapeutic approaches currently in fashion.

9.2　The Hippocratic healing tradition

In China, as well as in India and Greece, it appears that certain energetic circuits, such as the meridians, were discovered simultaneously. This knowledge was further cultivated and developed in India and China, whereas in Europe, it was to a large extent lost.

In the cradle of our Western culture and medicine, in Greece of the 5th century B.C., we find in the tradition of the doctor Hippocrates, in addition to the beginnings of somatic medicine, many important sources of a subtle energetic medicine and wisdom teaching. It was the objective of the followers of Hippocrates for the healing process to be shaped and harmonized. Here we can find keywords we currently use for our subtle energetic therapeutic applications: strengthen, delimit, reverse the polarity, drain, process, and structure. Every manifestation was experienced as a process, in other words, phases of a process corresponded to stages of consciousness, in contrast to Zen, for example, which is interested in intermediary stages as a means of accessing the spectrum of consciousness.

Rituals like marriage, fasting periods, and dying rituals were considered by the followers of Hippocrates to be structures – consciousness-expanding structures – in human life, as well as imparting structure in the case of an individual healing process. In every case, however, the theory, in Hippocrates' view, was oriented toward the patient's consciously formulated wish to change his life, in the sense of the Greek-Delphic γνῶθι σεαυτόν [gnothi seauton] = know thyself. It is Delphic because this sentence stood, as a "motto," over the entrance to the Temple of Apollo at Delphi, where the seer Pythia gave her prophecies.

It is true that much was written about Hippocrates, but – as we know since the studies of Annie Berner-Hürbin – it was probably written in coded form, such that here, ancient knowledge must be newly discovered in the truest sense of the word. Berner found code words in the ancient texts, and upon deciphering them, was able to translate them afresh, recognizing that they were actually ritual texts. Thus in the Hippocratic Oath, she sees the message that the consummation of healing action leads to spirituality. Healing – becoming healthy – is energetic development and can be experienced as a path.

It is not without significance that the genuine representatives of the healing methods centered around the Greek doctor Hippocrates were seers. Doctors who were not clairvoyant were considered to be charlatans, or in the best case, began to occupy themselves with somatic medicine, laboring merely technically and at a low level of knowledge and understanding. Whoever was afflicted with a surgical problem at the time was generally not very well attended to (as in the case of infections).

9.3 Different European healing traditions up to the middle of the 19th century

Western medicine owes much to the ancient Egyptians. Thousands of years ago, high-level healing methods and medicines were developed there. "A country full of doctors," noted the Greek Herodotus around 450 B.C. during his visit to Egypt. A part of this knowledge found its way via Greece to Europe.

The entire medical knowledge of his time was available to Aristotle, who was schooled among the Platonists, and he entrusted his pupil Menon with the task of methodically systematizing it. The Roman philosophers, too, including Cicero (106-43) and Seneca (4 B.C.-65 A.D.), possessed great knowledge of medicine. The connection between philosophical and therapeutic knowledge is also illustrated in the term used at the time: "iatro-sophist" (Greek ἰατρός [iatros] = doctor, σοφός [sophos] = wise man).[23] Claudius Galenus (129-199 A.D.) coined the familiar saying that a good doctor is (also) a good philosopher.

For us, too, the holistic healing approach is based on the idea that both the psyche and the body need to be healed, that one without the other is not possible, and that appropriately trained people need to be responsible for both components. The cultural achievement of Galen – personal physician to Roman Emperor Marcus Aurelius – was the systematization of the approximately 700 then-known healing plants according to their characteristics and their use as antidotes for illnesses. Galen was, nonetheless, already standing firmly in a tradition, able as he was to look back at the Ebers Papyrus, written 3500 years ago: a massive scroll 20 meters long that contained 800 pharmaceutical formulas. Galen's writings remained authoritatively connected with those of Hippocrates until well into the Middle Ages. This medical teaching was valid in Europe until the 19th century. It continues to be cultivated in monasteries to this day.

The European healing tradition subsequently underwent a change, since with the rise of Christianity, in addition to the mixture of the elements, the knowledge of healing plants, and the mystery cults, a significant force began to shape man: his soul, which he received as a gift from God. Someone who has a soul also has a mission in his life that must be fulfilled. According to the Christian religious teaching of sin and atonement, whoever strays from this path and risks failure becomes ill. Illness is now also understood as God's punishment. This concept takes its place next to the teaching of the elements, and from now on differentiates the European markedly from the Asian.

Illness, for the European Christian, is practically equated with the admission of one's lack of success. Healing is then a process of purification for the soul. This second aspect of the European healing tradition must not be neglected in subtle energetic treatments. The Asian forms of therapy, directed as they are primarily toward balance, do not incorporate this approach, still unconsciously of significance for the European.

In addition, we have the "witches' medicine." The healing knowledge of herb witches and monks certainly forms two important pillars in the tradition of European medicine. This herbal medicine is most likely a combination of specific knowledge from classical antiquity and other knowledge, much of which had been passed on orally for ages, mixed with Germanic-Celtic influences. The witches' approach of applying poison in small doses to heal illness eventually forms the basis for Hahnemann's homeopathy and the Anthroposophical medicine of Rudolf Steiner.

Practitioners of all of the ancient traditional healing methods were also familiar with the doctrine of signatures as used by primitive peoples: Creation communicates itself to the sick person through a sign (Lat. signum). For example, a plant that has kidney-shaped leaves could reveal itself to be a remedy for the kidneys. From our own experience, it is to be noted that the seed forms, above all, are instructive with regard to possible applications.

The first person who endeavored to raise the traditional stores of European knowledge in the medical domain, or the last person who carried this knowledge within himself, applying it successfully and developing it further, was the medieval doctor Paracelsus, whom we mentioned above. His most important insight was that there is a forming energy in man that extends beyond his life force. He called this immaterial principle **archeus** and meant by this the immortal soul. This shaping force is the fertile ground for success. According to Paracelsus, without referring to it, healing is impossible.

Fundamentally, we must add that from today's point of view, the original healing methods also attached great value to prophylaxis – already in Hippocratic healing medicine, the subject of diet was given much weight. When the ancient Chinese emperors fell ill, their doctors were dismissed, since the task of the doctor was to maintain the ruler's health. (Greek προ-φυλάσσω [prophylasso] = keep guard against something, protect oneself, prevent, and thus be vigilant in order to remain in equilibrium.)

In summary, we can say that up to the middle of the 19th century, people – including doctors – were aware of the infinite powers of man and his connection with the spiritual worlds and made conscious and active use of this. It was only later generations that disowned or were forced – whatever the reasons may have been – to disown the intuitive, living, and spiritual forces. The original holistic approach of the healing modalities was able to persist for a long time, well into the Roman and Christian era. Then through Byzantium, it was integrated into Arabic medicine and found entry into Europe once again via Spain. It finally appeared once more with the abbess Hildegard von Bingen, and produced, with Paracelsus, its last great representative.

Those practicing the traditional holistic healing arts healed the body through the soul. The domain of the soul, however, could not and cannot be proven by science. Ancient models of the soul correspond to a field theory. Academic science works with corpuscle theories.

It always seemed to us that our European tradition offered concepts of healing that were at least the equal of Chinese or Indian medicine, and that at the roots of our culture there is enough significant healing knowledge that can be built upon in a modern setting with bioenergetic healing experience and research. We are grateful in this regard for the valuable indications that provided substance to our conjecture and motivated us to continue testing and gathering personal experience. It seems reasonable to include the appropriate contributions of traditional healing knowledge in bioenergetic applications, in this way doing justice to today's European body in its healing process.

Subtle energetic healing was and is always anchored in society. Because they are rooted in society, the healing arts were at home in ritual healing and possibly also in the sacred and spiritual domains. In this sense, the healing arts are the image of a society and its mentality and spiritual orientation. Discovering ancient, subtle energetic healing knowledge is meaningful when it is correspondingly integrated into a society and its already existing medicine and has a fructifying effect on the body, soul, and spirit of man. Then resonance becomes therapy – and therapy resonance.

9.4 Practical model application of synchronous therapy using the Tensor and BIOSYN device

9.4.1 General description of the treatment

If life is communication, information, and resonance, then it is much more than the mere sum of chemical processes: It is the subtlest occurrence consisting of ceaseless activities in and between the most diverse cellular connections. All processes of life take place primarily in a microworld of vibrations and very diverse frequencies. The expression ν-έργεια [energeia] was also used by Plato for the exchange between human beings, among other things, and for the subtle perception of this exchange. Holistic healing and renewing health must include this interpersonal encounter, this being-touched (in the physical body and psyche).

If the quality of bioenergy sheds light on the information, communication, and resonance of the cells and organs among themselves, then with the Tensor we have a wonderful instrument for testing more than merely damage that has already physically manifested.

For this subtle energetic exchange and connectedness, the ancient Greeks used the expressions micro- and macrocosmos. In this age of scientific paradigm shift and multidimensionality, we use the more contemporary terms information, communication, and resonance, endeavoring to explore new therapeutic approaches through these terms and through the recognition of networkedness.

Let us try to rediscover the different levels of healing that have been lost, to include once again the subtle energetic aspects of healing, and to treat the oneness of body and soul. But let us do so in a form that corresponds to the development of our culture and our consciousness. We view such an understanding of the healing arts as an effective, necessary, and useful complement to academic medicine, the only form of medicine that had the chance to develop during the last centuries.

When by means of bioenergetic therapy, blocked energies are enabled to flow again, a lower quality of vibration is tuned to a higher one and an excess of energy is drained (or lack of energy is built up), a process of self-healing is set in motion, and helping us to help ourselves becomes an important theme.

Man's energetic bodies and energetic pathways (meridians) can be subtle energetically tested, described, and treated in advance. Naturally, an energetic diagnosis is important at the outset. A subtle energetic investigation with the Tensor, without further technical devices, includes systematically testing the basic energy, protective energy (immune system), glands, energetic pathways (meridians), the energy of individual organs, and if need be of the joints. Blood and urine testing then follows by means of polarity phases.

During the first examination, possible geopathic information regarding the body (location of bed) should always be determined as well. An evaluation of the teeth is then of great importance: The two principle energetic pathways of the human body (according to the Chinese healing tradition), the so-called Governing Vessel and Conception Vessel, end in the upper and lower palate, respectively. This suggests the degree to which energetic deficits and stimulation can be transmitted from the oral cavity throughout the entire body, and inversely, how pain (often incomprehensible to the dentist) can manifest in the teeth through organic afflictions.

Although practiced testers will not conjure up laboratory values for the thyroid and pancreas, for example, they can almost instantaneously (and affordably!) detect disorders connected to excessive or insufficient function – even individually for the exocrine and endocrine[24] areas of the pancreas – present already in the subtle energetic domain, and can supply them with energetically positive information, in other words, react before damage becomes clinically manifest. In the subtle energetic domain, stresses on the body due to amalgam fillings (mercury), environmental poisons, electrosmog, etc., can be systemically tested extremely quickly.

Experience shows, however, that illness approaches the body through many different vibrational levels. We can picture these different levels like concentric circles surrounding our body. In this way, subtle energetic harm that is not yet demonstrable through laboratory values in conventional medicine, can be treated and eliminated. Incidentally, an ailment departs from the body in the same way, only in reverse: Illness often withdraws slowly through the different energetic levels (from the level close to the body up to more subtle vibrational levels) until it disappears. This is the reason why it is possible to subtle energetically test whether a healing process is proceeding correctly, even when clinically, no changes are (as yet) discernible.

Vertebral column tests are also interesting and informative. It has often happened that through dysfunctions tested in the vertebral column, holistic correlations to poorly functioning organs could be made, or ill people could be referred to other, more useful therapies since, for example, a vertebra first needed to be adjusted. Indeed, the painful area is often not the area that is truly ill. The latter can be found with the Tensor, in this way providing a useful indication to therapists who may otherwise be at a loss.

Initial examinations should not be carried out without testing glasses, jewelry, watches, piercings, amulets, and so on. Food intolerances should also be questioned and tested. Moreover, we have an excellent opportunity to eliminate or improve allergies with subtle energetic treatment methods. During the first examination, the client should bring along any allopathic medications he may be taking; they should be tested by means of a relational test to the client, and the individual medications should then be tested in relation to each other. If such medications are not compatible with one another, or if they reveal themselves to be incompatible with the client, one should confer with the prescribing doctor. There are so many medications nowadays that it is usually possible to find a compatible combination. According to the client's objective and type, the chakras – the body's subtlest energetic vortices – can be tested. In this way, a holistic picture gradually emerges of the client's energetic state, with respect to both his psyche and his physical body.

As is well known, health is more than the absence of illness. Health is the perfect communication between the cells, the harmonic interplay of all our organs, glands, nerves, and senses, and ultimately of our body, soul, and spirit. If this harmony falls out of equilibrium, first the feeling of being unwell appears and later illness makes itself known. **We defined bioenergy as a carrier of messages, a carrier of information, and thus, we could say, a carrier of information about the metabolism, in short: about life.**

Once the bioenergetic energy diagnosis of a client, that is, the information about his state of health, is available to us, it is also advisable to introduce other vibrational information by means of a bioenergetic treatment. Such a form of therapy has the goal of bringing about a balanced equilibrium in the body's subtle energies, such as the harmonious functioning of the glandular and hormonal system, or the possible regulation of the enzyme and mineral metabolism. This, together with inner equilibrium, is what ensures health in the organism.

With regard to its spectrum and intensity of action, the BIOSYN device is comparable to more elaborately equipped electronic devices. The BIOSYN device does not use the electric circuit, working instead with rechargeable batteries. The effectiveness of this device is based on a principle that does not require any electricity. It is small and easy to use, which is very practical for therapy with animals (including unconfined animals), landscapes, trees, plants, and bodies of water. It cannot and does not intend to give computerlike indications, since in such a case, in our view, the word bioresonance would be brought to the point of absurdity. The device was tested on different trips and with different travel complaints, including a very striking experience in the desert, where it was possible to work successfully with only one's own vibration (where could an electrical outlet or computer be found?). In order to be able to make full use of the device with all its facets and possibilities, corresponding training is necessary.

Fundamentally, the device offers three intra-device-generated frequencies: harmonizing, sedating, and vitalizing. It also works with reverse vibrations (inverse vibrations) which can be used following anesthesia, lengthy treatments with antibiotics or cortisone, and with allergies, to cite a few examples. In addition, tested substances (vibrational substances) can be entered and stored as external reference values.

Since the BIOSYN device does not work according to the laws of classical homeopathy or phytotherapy, exploring instead new therapeutic paths in the field of vibrational medicine, a different spectrum of therapies is, to a certain extent, available for use here than is usually the case – also in classical bioresonance. This type of informational and vibrational therapy, which we refer to as **synchronous therapy**, has not yet been truly described. It can be best understood through the books of James L. Oschman, Manfred Doepp, and of Annie Berner-Hürbin in its more extended philosophical sense.[25]

Examples of the application of basic settings:

HARMONIZING: It is a fact that the bioenergy of a patient who has undergone surgery is not located on his body, but at least one meter away from it. Through the mediation of harmonizing vibrations, the bioenergy is brought back to the body; thus providing the patient with a clearly better feeling, as well as a better, and above all, shorter healing process.

SEDATING: This vibrational action can be used for all inflammatory processes, as well as for hyper reactions of organs and glands (for example, hyperthyroidism).

TONIFYING: Stimulating energetic vibration in cases of immune weakness or other states of weakness in individual organs or glands, joints, etc.

INFORMATION: A tested external reference value can, potentiated 1:1 or by 100 times, be introduced into the organism or applied isopathically as a self-vibration.

SYNCHRONIZING: Pathological vibrations can be eliminated and reversed. Here one must be careful not to eliminate the action of any long-term medications prescribed by a doctor (such as blood pressure medications, etc.).

An example of therapy for a bee sting: The upper arm swells to almost twice its normal size, although there is no known allergy. With the reverse setting (mirroring), subsequent harmonization and the vibrational introduction of homeopathic Apis, the arm swelling is gone in a day. It would also be possible here to treat using the afflicted arm's own energy (= isopathic treatment).

It is an imperative necessity to check and supervise the entire treatment process and progression with the Tensor. Not only the treatment modalities, but also the intensity and length of vibrational introduction, extraction, or neutralization must be tested in order to guarantee an optimal application. Once the treatment has been concluded, the client should present good overall energy, and all tested points, meridians, organs, etc., should vibrate with the same intensity. The frequency with which such applications must be repeated is determined according to the individual and the illness, and possibly according to a calendar date tested with the Tensor.

Synchronous therapy has never been understood as an alternative to conventional medicine, but as complementary to it, not least because each client is tested individually (without a computer), as are the corresponding use of the device and vibrational applications when necessary. In our experience, informational and energetic medicine is very much a **cost-saving** medicine, for which the time is long overdue: Hospital stays cannot always be avoided, but they can be shortened, and the use of medications can be minimized when medication combinations, as well as the time of day and quantity to be taken, are tested. Using the Tensor optimizes the choice of medications, their interaction, and their dosage.

A woman in her mid-80s was hospitalized due to an emergency: a case of acute heart insufficiency. On her way to the bathroom at night, she fell several times, resulting in two black eyes, broken ribs, and a lung infection. The dizziness she experienced at night was not given any attention – it was ascribed to her age. A choice of two heart medications was available to the specialist – the plan was to try them out. With the Tensor it was attempted to test for the right heart medication, as well as the necessary combination of the entire chemical cocktail. The lady never fell again. In the package leaflet of the wrongly administered medication, it was noted that it could cause dizziness. If someone had been able to test the two available medications at the hospital, the woman (and the health insurance company) would have been spared more than two months' hospital stay. It is to be noted that none of the doctors could have known which would have been the appropriate medication.

In general, the medications that are tested and are in resonance with the client can be of any origin. They often clearly indicate to the tester the vibrational plane into which the healing process should be directed. In agreement with the ancient healing traditions, it is our opinion that even people who are physically healthy would benefit by undergoing a subtle energetic test/treatment as a matter of prevention two to three times a year, very much in the spirit of the ancient Chinese emperors – and certainly also due to the cost explosion in the field of disease prevention.

Our experience over many years shows that remnants of former illnesses, illnesses considered by conventional medicine to be "taken care of," are still testable at an informational level and thus represent a lifelong burden to our "vibrational baggage." The vibration (information) of an illness can be more harmful in the long term than the illness itself during its acute phase. Here as well, the non-visible is often more important than the visible. These are some of the insights of energetic and informational medicine. Any old information that can be neutralized increases our fundamental health potential – and this type of treatment, understandably, works best for otherwise healthy people.

It is understandable that a healthy body that receives the subtlest resonant impulses through the medium of water, for example, progresses in its inner process – if it so desires – in the sense of "becoming who you are." Through the body's water, we can detect the minutest energetic imbalances, which the client himself may not yet have physically noticed at all. Generally speaking, through a treatment using the BIO-SYN device – above all in connection with water therapy – a process is initiated that manifests itself not only somatically, but often even more markedly at the level of the psyche. This pattern of application also corresponds to the insight of eternally flowing energies and continually alternating process phases. In this way, our human energetic potential can be developed, since each phase carries within itself the potential of transformation.

It is not the therapist who determines the type of treatment, unless he is intuitive and clairvoyant like the Hippocratic doctors. We have the Tensor, which informs us about our system of testing, as well as the level of healing, vibrational fields, and resonance remedies to be worked with. The affliction in question can be at a coarsely material level, but it can also require energetic support of the chakras or strengthening of the aura. In every case, it is important for the therapist to have sufficiently broad medical knowledge so that in appropriate situations, medical examinations and clarifications can be recommended in a timely manner.

The breathing rhythm, as transitional phenomenon between body and psyche and as carrier of subtle energies, should also be mentioned here. During synchronous therapy, people and animals begin to breathe differently, with at least one deep inhale…most easily observed in horses and dogs.

As an accompaniment to other therapies, informational, energetic medicine can have an optimizing action, for example during chemotherapy or radiation therapy for cancer patients. Subtle energetic treatments of pregnant women are touching: Once a month, healthy pregnant women are optimally supplied energetically on an individual basis, through healing water and flowers. The effect is physical well-being and inner balance – apparently for the baby as well. According to all reports, the behavior of these infants is calmer and more balanced from the very beginning.

Bioenergetically, the burdens of these arriving souls can evidently be lightened to a certain extent.

In the context of our concept of energy transmission, the person giving the treatment must be aware that negative elements could be transferred; therefore it is necessary for him to actively examine his ethical attitude and his state of health. "In purity and according to divine law..."

Knowledge of the importance of polarity in the human body and the recognition of its possibilities for testing have greatly enriched the types of bioenergetic applications in the human body, and restoration of the correct polarity in the appropriate location has already brought about striking improvements in health. Every polarity is a tension that gives rise to movement.

In ancient Greek medicine in the tradition of the doctor Hippocrates, one of the goals was to clairvoyantly perceive the right moment of time for the treatment, namely the moment in time which – whatever the reasons may be – represents a synchronous moment in which therapist (operator) and patient form a subtle interference pattern. καιρός [kairos] = the (right) moment in time. With the Tensor, we have the possibility of testing, if we wish to do so, data for operative interventions or other therapies. Both doctors and dentists who perform their academic work along with subtle energetic knowledge have confirmed to us their positive results in this regard.

9.4.2 Water treatment

In combination with the BIOSYN device, we have developed a special application within the context of our bioenergetic water research. The BIOSYN device offers a particular spectrum of application in this area. Through the electrodes, it is able to energetically improve any type of water, both in the bathtub and the water jug. The improvement here does not take place at the coarse, technical level, but only by means of subtle vibrations, in such a way that energetically speaking, water treated with the BIOSYN device is similar to the water that flows around primary rocks. It has been shown to be optimal to connect the device to the water tap in order to remove stress from the tap water and to enable us to consume shower, bath, and cooking/drinking water that has the vibrational quality of such "primary rock" water. When this is done, swimming pools and biotopes need to be treated with significantly fewer chemicals. By harmonizing all the water pipes in a building, the basic energy is also improved in one's living space, house, and workplace.

Through our insights into the characteristics specific to water, we have developed, in connection with our practical device, our own water application. The point of departure was the idea that it could be an effective treatment concept for 70-80% of the human body – that is, its entire water component – to be brought into a specific healing vibration. Through individually and vibrationally informed water, we are usually able to observe a considerable effect on both the psychological and physical domains, a profound change in a person's state of health at the juncture of body and soul. We have thus recorded successes with exogenous forms of depression (mourning, workplace harassment, divorce); with psychological disorientation in life (a frequent phenomenon of our times); as an application that improves the quality of life and strengthens the immune system in patients undergoing chemotherapy and radiation therapy; as a subtle energetic accompaniment during pregnancy; and with blood disease.

Through water therapy, it is possible to learn much about a person's state of health. Recognition and understanding of the principle of resonance incites us to be particularly careful during treatment of infants, the elderly, and very sick and weakened people, as well as pregnant women. Experience shows that there are bodily states in which the body is so blocked or weakened that it no longer follows the principles of resonance. For this reason, the basics of water applications are also tested on people directly, foregoing electronic devices and schematic treatment procedures.

9.4.3 Isopathic application

A further interesting treatment possibility is offered by the isopathic principle. Isopathic treatments occupy an important place in the context of our bioenergetic applications and research. Our grandmothers had no knowledge of chemical insecticide sprays for the pests found on their plants at home and in the garden. They added lice to the water used for watering that had been left to sit for a certain amount of time, ideally under the sun. Afterwards, this informed water was poured on the affected plants – and usually with success. Paracelsus, too, recommended drawing out a poison with the same poison – it is all only a matter of the dosage.

Today isopathic remedies are commercially available; they contain the same pathogenic strain as the bacteria itself, for example, with the only difference that it is homeopathically "diluted." An isopathic healing results in an avoidance of side-effects in the body and the elimination of harmful microbes.

To truly remain in the subtle energetic domain, we usually work, however, with the body's pathological subtle energy, which we collect and introduce again, in potentiated form, into the corresponding organism. An extremely effective treatment method is the testing of remedies that are resonant with the pathological vibration, which often provides, on the intellectual level, an explanation of the as yet unknown pathology to the experienced practitioner. This type of vibrational isopathic treatment has demonstrated itself to be extremely effective above all for plants and animals – and here it is not possible to speak of a placebo effect.

Nero the dog is brought in for treatment with a benign but inoperable tumor. It is inoperable because it is too close to his eye. For this reason he is treated only isopathically through the tumor's own vibration, and for three days he passes urine constantly. One hour before the planned trip to the veterinarian, the urination subsides and the tumor melts, disappearing completely and definitively.

9.4.4 Harmonizing vibrations for the dying process

Experience has shown that a dying person, at a particular point in time, no longer has any resonance with remedies, and possibly harmonizing energies or flowers and scents, helpful to the dying process. In ancient Greece, no more attempts at healing were made when the patient could in truth no longer be saved. Knowledge of the silver cord, which holds the body and soul together, most likely still existed at the time and consequently also the knowledge that when this silver cord becomes loose, remedies are no longer appropriate.

In humans and animals, the body's energy diminishes progressively during the dying process; what is happening is the gradual extinguishing of the biophotons' ultracoherent light. Bioenergetic devices display, at most, harmonizing frequencies. It is also possible, through ignorance, to make the passage at the subtle energetic level more difficult. Bioenergy is produced by metabolism (for example). When metabolism becomes slower, the quantity of bioenergy is also reduced. This is one of the explanations why, in the process of dying, any resonance with remedies can no longer be tested.

A dying person who, at his own request, is being accompanied by healing water applications, describes the process as follows: "All the different energetic and vibrational circles are closing around me in an ordered and concentric way. I'm coming into an unbelievable harmony; I'm coming into my center." Fifteen minutes after I left, the person passed away.

To the astonishment of the professional bird care station, we were able – with our method and much patience – to raise Fipsli, a starling, from just a few days old until he was fully fledged. While he was in the house learning to fly, Fipsli broke his neck. We informed the dying little bird with harmonizing energy, during which something unbelievable happened: His little hanging head started moving and straightened on his body – a liberating chirp and the bird was dead. It is good to witness such an event when you are not alone, in order to be certain of what you have seen.

Harmonizing vibrations can have their value not only for living, but also for dying. Corresponding energetic measures are useful when **physical healing is no longer possible** and the therapist, with respect for life, is called upon to facilitate the person's passing on.

The possibility of testing bioenergy, as a carrier of information, on living beings gives rise to a new – and also ethically new – approach to the discussion about abortion, organ transplantation, and euthanasia.

9.5 Summary

Through the different treatment procedures that have been tested, the cells, the body's water, and the organs are informed through synchronous therapy in such a way that they are able to better communicate again and to find their resonance partners. Synchronous therapy has the goal of inciting the biophotons of the sick cells to a resonant and networked exchange of light once again. In healing processes that are set in motion by subtle energy, energies and information promoting order are transmitted to the sick organism. The exchange of light among cells observed by Fritz-Albert Popp in the light intensifier he developed can be detected by the Tensor, through an intensive up-and-down oscillation. The type of treatment described above includes the initial energetic diagnosis of the energy field emanating from the living creature, as well as its energetic use for therapeutic applications, followed by instrument-based amplification of natural, subtle energetic, external signals, and electromagnetic information.

Following many years of bioenergetic tests on the human body, we can accept that the human organism truly does form a coherent (holographic) electromagnetic field which, however, extends beyond the boundaries of the body. The water in a person's body also transmits information far away from the body (cf. Chapter 8). In this way, we find an explanation for the human aura, spoken of by clairvoyants for millennia, as well as for the electromagnetic fields measured by Poltyakov, Korotkov, and others.

How is it possible, then, that energy fields, widely known as they were in earlier civilizations, continue to be largely unknown in our latitudes, and interest in them stamped as "esoteric" in the negative sense, taboo for normal thinkers? People practicing traditional holistic healing arts in all the ancient advanced civilizations healed the body, by means of energy fields, through the soul. What belongs to the domain of the soul, however, cannot be proven by science. Energetic informational medicine, with its subjectivity and to a large extent continued immeasurability in the traditional scientific sense, does not by any means render the laws of rationality and the status quo of contemporary medicine inoperative. Subtle energetic treatments can **enhance** what is attained by contemporary medicine in border and problem areas with important aspects and vibrational levels (above all through the domain of the psyche or soul).

Synchronous therapy, developed by Norbert Seiler and extended further by ourselves, has the goal of strengthening the dissipative system of humans, animals, and plants in such a way that they are capable, even in today's more difficult conditions (environment, stress, electrosmog, etc.), of integrating everything new that continually presents itself, receiving benefit from what is new and eliminating what is old and unusable (including old vibrational patterns from past illnesses or medicinal therapies) – similar to water in nature, which renews itself while naturally flowing over the stones of the river bed and casting off negative information. The moment a permeable system is no longer able to accommodate change, it is blocked and cuts itself off from the vitality of life.

Since bioenergy – as we have shown – is defined and understood by us as a carrier of information, and thus provides clues about information, communication, the quality of resonance, and the healthy networkedness of the cells and organs, it is for us a legitimate and useful ancient healing modality that we are endeavoring to implement in an appropriately contemporary manner. With the Tensor as testing instrument, we hold fast to the principle and our conviction, that testing and healing should once again be done more directly on the person, rather than through an apparatus.

The dissemination and growing acceptance of subtle energetic treatment methods is encouraging. The extent to which booming technical-apparatus medicine will really have a relation to subtle energy, however, is questionable. The aim is not for a "bioenergetic conventional medicine" to be developed, but rather for the particularities of informational and energetic medicine to be accepted and integrated. Making vibrations visible, the understanding of modern (meta-) physics, and the great wealth of positive experience may be enough, at some point, for acceptance. With the paradigm shift, the era in which there existed only the academic measuring stick is over. For a holistic alternative medicine, however, comprehensive knowledge of the physical, mental, and spiritual levels are a precondition: healing as a path of development.

Those for whom the new "old awareness" of the field theories of current physics is becoming a reality will no longer need to engage in therapeutic arguments or justifications. They will see themselves as embedded in the ancient healing arts of our Western tradition.

"The universe is far more complex and coherent than anyone other than poets and mystics have dared to imagine."
Ervin László

10. CONCLUSION

About 30 years ago, we began testing and researching bioenergy and bioenergetic phenomena, as well as working with bioenergetic applications in the area of health. Much has changed since then. What was seen at the time to be strange New Age ideas is today – as we have shown – taken seriously by scientists, and above all described in physics and metaphysics, and seen by them as at least a possible model of thought, if not heralded under the banner of paradigm shift as the newly discovered reality. What pioneers in the medical field attempted to implement at the time from the first insights of bioresonance therapy – and were scoffed at – is today, under the title of informational and energetic medicine, practiced and described by some conventional medical practitioners.

We have always believed that knowledge of the essence and action of subtle bioenergy can serve to optimize our quality of life in an increasingly compromised environment (water, food, living location), as well as serve as an optimizing complement in all areas of healing. We have always been convinced that research and education are necessary in this field. Bioenergy is life energy. Who has ever heard anything about this at school?

If we have succeeded in awakening in readers a curiosity about our life energy's principle of action, about the beneficial implementation of the ancient knowledge of this principle in our current era, and in convincing them of the necessity of including knowledge of bioenergy in everyday life, nature (environmental protection), and healing practice, we have accomplished our goal. May many people be able to improve their everyday lives and health by applying this knowledge.

Resonance, information, communication. These three concepts define life. They are fundamental ordering principles in which the cosmos and our life pulsate and function. In this respect, everything we do must be oriented to these principles. When we attend to these laws and deal with them knowingly, life does not become easier, it is true, but it does become more harmonious, explainable, and can be shaped more meaningfully.

ACKNOWLEDGMENTS

It remains for me to thank the people who contributed to the genesis of this work. First of all, my two daughters: Nathalie, who not only guided me "electronically," and attentively and critically accompanied the text in progress, but also worked tirelessly in every possible way for the work's publication; and Eliane, who formulated fundamental objections, ideas, and questions during the initial phase. Thank you to my husband Heinz, who encouraged me for years to write this book.

I would like to thank three friends: In memoriam of my dear friend Marianne Engeler-Merz, who passed away too early and whom, as a competent discussion partner and stimulating sharer of ideas for many years, I miss very much; Brigitte von Rechenberg for her coherent and friendly introduction; and both her and Regula Sauerländer for their human accompaniment, encouragement, and valuable conversations about the subject.

For everything relating to ancient Greek spellings and textual passages, I was advised by classical philologist Hansjörg Vogel, for which I express my gratitude. The expert illustrations in this book were done by Maeva Arnold and Jacques Laesser. A warm thank you to Silvia Pfisterer and Andrea Vock, who made several photographs available to me. Thank you also for the sensitive editing of the English version by Janice Geiser, Aarau.

I express my thanks to all the medical people who, from early on, took our work seriously and even noticed it, supporting us by securing, for example, laboratory test values, in short: were not afraid of joint patient-client care.

ENDNOTES

[1] Taubes, G., (1984). *Die Geburt der Schneeflocken.* Tages Anzeiger Magazin Nr. 7.

[2] Today working together at BIONIK AG. www.bionik-ag.ch.

[3] The terms **eidos, energeia,** and **enetelecheia** appear countless times in passages from Aristotle. The lines between these concepts are often blurred. This characteristic of using several synonymous terms for something very specific was already present in Plato. Aristotle Metaphys. 8.1045b: Energy-Dynamis; Metaphys. 11.1065b-1066a: Dynamis-Entelechy-Energy; Metaph.8.1042a: Energy-Dynamis.

[4] In the most ancient traditions of all cultures there can be found descriptions of the seven whirling electromagnetic fields (Indian "chakras") of the human body, which together create our aura and which can be characterized as centers of consciousness of the energetic or etheric body.

[5] The so-called Einstein-Podolsky-Rosen-Paradox (1935) states that there can be correlations between systems that are spatially far away from each other, correlations that cannot be explained through direct interaction. Further experiments (Alain Aspect, 1982) showed that the two systems must not be regarded as separate systems at all, but as a unity. And if they form a unity, we can no longer speak of a transmission of information.

[6] Korotkov, K. (1999). *Aura and Consciousness: New stage of scientific understanding.* Russian Ministry of Culture St. Petersburg.

[7] When the test person can resist the pressure from the outside on his wrist (with his arm held outward), he tests "strong," that is, he is not negatively influenced by the test stimulus. If he cannot resist the

pressure, he tests "weak," that is, his life energy is negatively influenced by the test stimulus. More detailed instructions and information about the muscle test are contained in the book, Diamond, J., *Your Body Doesn't Lie*. Sydney: Harper & Row, 1979.

8   The expression **entelechy** consists of the three syllables en, tel, and echeia: ἐν [en] = in, τέλος [telos] = goal, echeia from ἔcein [echein] = have, so it firstly means a goal-oriented action or activity. With Aristotle, it meant something that has its goal in itself, form that realizes itself in matter, the active principle that transforms the possible into reality. For Aristotle, "ὕλη [hyle] = matter without εἶδος [eidos] = form only has possibility and no reality, while form is the actualizing factor that bestows reality and is thus the goal of the process of becoming. Aristotle uses entelechy nearly synonymously with energy.

9   According to Paracelsus (1493-1541) – by his real name Philipp Aureolus Theophrastus Bombastus von Hohenheim – the inner person consists of a nonmaterial life principle, the "archeus." This life force or "spiritual essence," which is present everywhere but invisible – though of etheric substance, a substance nonetheless – remains bound to the body as long as it dwells in it. It departs from the body at the moment of death. In a state of health, the archeus is equally distributed throughout all parts of the body. One could say it is the invisible nourishment from which the visible body draws its force. A doctor who neglects this life force is, according to Paracelsus, nothing more than a quack. Cf. on this subject: Hartmann, F. (1891). *The life and the doctrines of Paracelsus.*

10 Driesch, Hans, (1909). *Die Philosophie des Organischen.* Verlag Quelle & Meyer Leipzig.

11 In our current age, the world of physics is still divided. Some physicists are searching for a new world view, while another group is searching for a "world formula" that would sweep away all problems and confirm – at least on the most general level – the current world

view. The third, and probably largest group does not concern itself with the philosophical aspects of quantum physics. It makes use of the approaches of quantum physics in order to develop new technical possibilities, and ignores everything that, on the basis of its world view, is not supposed to exist.

[12] Verband für Radiästhesie und Geobiologie Schweiz (Swiss Association for Radiesthesia and Geobiology), 9010 St. Gallen, President René Näf.

[13] Faraday Cage: an encasement of a room on all sides, made out of lead or wire netting, for the purpose of shielding against external electric and magnetic fields. Cars, planes, and the wire system of a lightning conductor installation surrounding a building, are Faraday Cages. (Michael Faraday, English physicist, 1791-1867). In a Faraday Cage, the Tensor indicates a zero, that is, no bioenergy – thus the fatigue we experience, for example, after a long car trip.

[14] Nonetheless: in the Series for Environmental Protection No. 98, the summary reads: "Laboratory and field investigations show that biosystems can be disrupted by non-ionizing electromagnetic radiation according to intensity, frequency, means of radiation, and length of exposure." What does the press tell us today about this?
Der Einfluss von nichtionisierender elektromagnetischer Strahlung auf die Umwelt (The influence of non-ionizing electromagnetic radiation on the environment). Edited by the Federal Office for Environmental Protection, Bern, December 1988.

[15] Bovis Biometer: measure to radiesthetically determine the energetic intensity of a location, person, or thing, developed by the French physicist Bovis. For example, the physical energy of a healthy person measures 6500 Bovis units.

[16] My Lord and my God,
take everything from me
that keeps me from Thee.

My Lord and my God,
give everything to me
that brings me near to Thee.

My Lord and my God,
take me away from myself
and give me completely to Thee.

Amen

[17] Curry, M, Dr. med.,(1978). *Curry-Netz*, Herold-Verlag, Verlag Dr.Wetzel und Co., Munich.
Hartmann, E., Dr. med., (1976). *Krankheit als Standortsproblem*, Haug-Verlag, Heidelberg.
Endrös, Robert, (1978). *Die Strahlung der Erde*, Paffrath Verlag Remscheid.
Mettler, M.L.,(1986). *Atmosphärische Reizstreifen*, Metaphysik 2000, Moser, Verlag CH-Zürich.

[18] Pogačnik, M., (1989). *Die Erde Heilen*, Eugen Diederichs Verlag München.
Website: www.hagia-chora.org.

[19] "Ether, the vacuum field, zero-point energy, the scalar field, and implicit order are not foreign and unconnected to the theory of biophotons, but implicitly contained in it… […] Perhaps the coherent carrier wave field, which Popp characterizes as potential information, originates in a kind of vacuum state."
Bischof, M., (1995). *Biophotons, the Light in our Cells*, Verlag Zweitausendundeins Frankfurt a. Main, p.163.

[20] Broadband noise: For an energy exchange, all that is needed are very weak signals, which even with modern measuring equipment are lost in so-called noise. For this reason they cannot be scientifically proven.

[21] For example:
Lauterwasser, A., (2002). *Wasser Klang Bilder,* AT Verlag Aarau.
Emoto, M., (2000). *The Message from Water,* Hado.
Bischof, M., Op.cit.p.310: *Das Gedächtnis des Wassers.*

[22] Translated by Michael North, National Library of Medicine, 2002.

[23] Lichtenthaeler, Ch. (1984). *Der Eid des Hippokrates. Ursprung und Bedeutung.* Deutscher Aerzte-Verlag Cologne p. 90.

[24] Endocrine (Gr.): with inner secretion, that is, delivering into the blood (hormonal glands).
Exocrine (Gr.): with secretion toward the outside (salivary glands, sweat glands etc.).

[25] Doepp, M., (2008). *Energie und Kosmos. Die Medizin des 21.Jahrhunderts.* COMED Verlagsgesellschaft GmbH Hochheim.
Oschman, J. L. (2006). *Energiemedizin. Konzepte und ihre wissenschaftliche Basis.* Urban und Fischer Verlag Munich.
Berner-Hürbin, A., (1997). *Hippokrates und die Heilenergie. Alte und neue Modelle für eine holistische Therapeutik.* Schwabe und Co. AG Verlag Basel.

FURTHER LITERATURE

Banzhaf, D. et al., (1992). *Den ganzen Menschen heilen. Gesund werden. Gesund bleiben.* Verlag Stiftung Gralsbotschaft Stuttgart.

Berner-Hürbin, A., (1997). *Hippokrates und die Heilenergie.* Verlag Schwabe und Co. AG Basel.

Bischof, M.,. (1995). *Biophotonen, Das Licht in unsern Zellen.* Verlag Zweitausendundeins Frankfurt am Main.

Bischof M., (2002). *Tachionen, Orgonenergie, Skalarwellen, Feinstoffliche Felder zwischen Mythos und Wissenschaft.* AT Verlag Aarau.

Bösch, J., *Spirituelles Heilen und Schulmedizin.* AT Verlag Aarau.

Capra, F. (1975). *The Tao of Physics.* Shambhala Publications.

Capra, F., (1982). *The Turning Point: Science, Society, and the Rising Culture.* Simon and Schuster.

Capra, F., (1987). *Uncommon Wisdom: Conversations with Remarkable People.* Simon and Schuster.

Davis, J. S., (1995). *Ist Wasser mehr als H20? Das Lebenselement zwischen Mythos und Molekül.* Vortragsreihe „pantha rhei" der Hans Erni-Stiftung Luzern, Band XVI. Verlag Hans Erni Stiftung Luzern.

Devereux, P., (1992). *Earth Memory: Sacred Sites – Doorways into Earth's Mysteries.* Llewellyn Publications.

Diamond, J., (1979). *Your Body Doesn't Lie.* Harper & Row, Sydney.

Doepp, Manfred, (2008). *Energie und Kosmos, Die Medizin des 21.*

Jahrhunderts. Edition CO-MED. Verlagsgesellschaft GmbH Hochheim.

Emoto, M., (2000). *The Message of Water.* Hado.

Emoto, M., (2007). *The Shape of Love: Discovering Who We Are, Where We Came From, and Where We Are Going.* Doubleday, New York.

Endrös, R., (1978). *Die Strahlung der Erde.* Paffrath Verlag Remscheid.

Free B. & Dr. Hynaar (2001). *HAARP, Mindcontrol und wissenschaftlicher Irrsinn.* Pantha Rheo Verlag Wadern.

Curry, M. (1978). *Curry-Netz, das Reaktionsliniensystem als krankheitsauslösender Faktor,* Gesammelte Aufsätze, Herold-Verlag Dr.Wetzel München-Solln.

Grof, S., (2005). *When the Impossible Happens: Adventures in Non-Ordinary Reality.* Sounds True.

Hachenay, W., (1992). *WASSER, ein Gast der Erde.* Dingfelder-Verlag Andechs.

Kalbermatten, R., (2002). *Wesen und Signatur der Heilpflanzen.* AT Verlag Aarau.

Krug, A., (1993). *Heilkunst und Heilkult, Medizin in der Antike.* Verlag C. H. Beck München.

Laszlo, E. (2003). *The Connectivity Hypothesis: Foundations of an Integral Science of Quantum, Cosmos, Life, and Consciousness.* State University of New York Press.

Lauterwasser, A., (2002) *Wasser-Klang-Bilder.* Die schöpferische Musik des Weltalls. AT-Verlag Aarau.

Lauterwasser, A., (2005). *Wasser Musik, Geheimnis und Schönheit im Zusammenspiel von Wasser und Klangwellen.* AT-Verlag Baden und München.

Leadbeater, C.W., (1927). *The Chakras.* Theosophical Publishing House, Wheaton, Illinois.

Mayer / Winklbaur, (1986). *Biostrahlen. Der Mensch im Strahlungsfeld von Kosmos, Erde und Umwelt.* Verlag ORAC Wien.

Merz, B., (1984). *Orte der Kraft.* Institut de Recherches en Geobiologie Chardonne.

Merz, B., (1989). *Orte der Kraft in der Schweiz.* AT Verlag, Aarau.

Merz, B., (2000). *Die Seele des Ortes,* AT Verlag Aarau.

Mettler, M. L. (1986). *Atmosphärische Reizstreifen. Das Mass-System antiker Völker.* Moser Verlag Zürich.

Oschmann, J. L., (2006). *Energiemedizin. Konzepte und ihre wissenschaftliche Basis.* Urban und Fischer Verlag München.

Pennick N. (1995) *The Ancient Science of Geomancy: Living in Harmony with the Earth.* CRCS Publications.

Pogačnik, M., (1989). *Die Erde heilen.* Eugen Diederichs Verlag München.

Popp, F. A. (1999) *Die Botschaft unserer Nahrung.* Verlag Zweitausendundeins Frankfurt.

Rieger B., (2005). *Traditionelle Europäische Medizin, Heilkunst und Rezepte der Mönche und Kräuterhexen*. Verlag Herbig GmbH München.

Schwenk, T., (1974). *Das sensible Chaos: Strömendes Formenschaffen in Wasser und Luft*. Verlag Berlag Freies Geistesleben Stuttgart.

Sheldrake, R., (1981). *A New Science of Life: the hypothesis of formative causation*. J.P. Tarcher, Los Angeles.

Sheldrake, R., (1988). *The Presence of the Past: morphic resonance and the habits of nature*. Times Books, New York.

Tomkins, P. & C. Bird, (1989). *The Secret Life of Plants*. Harper & Row.

Von Bingen, H., (1994), *Heilwissen. Von den Ursachen und der Behandlung von Krankheiten*. Herder Verlag Freiburg im Breisgau.

Wetzel, C. M. (1976). *Radiästhesie - Rute und Pendel - heute*. Herold-Verlag Verlag Dr. Wetzel München.

ABOUT THE AUTHOR

Irene Zweifel-Lanz studied Romance languages and literature in Zurich, Lisbon, and Madrid from 1969 to 1974. From 1973 to 1978, she taught at various secondary schools. During this time she was also active as a journalist for the culture section of the *Neue Zürcher Zeitung* and as a translator.

In 1985 she began her training in the field of bioenergy in Kirchzarten, Germany. Between 1991 and 1994, she was trained as a registered German naturopath at the Isolde Richter School in Kenzingen, Germany. Further FMH Swiss Medical Association training followed on the subjects of "The Hippocratic Tradition and Science of Healing," "The Hippocratic Tradition and Socratic Psychotherapy," and a seminar on "Subtle Energetic Communication" with Dr. phil. Annie Berner-Hürbin.

She is currently active with BIONIK AG in the fields of Informational and Energy Medicine and as a seminar leader. The author lives in Aarau, Switzerland, is married and is the mother of two adult daughters.

Previously published works by the author:
"Open Letter to Pepe España." In: Dr. A. Röthlisberger (Ed.), *Pepe España Pintor.* (pp. 51-58). Buscho Buchdruckereien Schöftland AG, 1994.

"Jean-Pierre Monnier. The Universe of the Novel as Metaphor for the Search for Meaning." In: J. Bättig and S. Leimgruber (Eds.), *Grenzfall Literatur, die Sinnfrage in der modernen Literatur der viersprachigen Schweiz.* (pp. 681-693). Universitätsverlag & Paulusverlag Freiburg, 1993.

"Awakening to a New Language, Awakening to a New Being: Basic Themes and Leitmotifs in the Work of Jean-Pierre Monnier." In: Prof. Dr. J. Olbert & Dr. U. Wielandt (Eds.), *Französisch heute. Jubiläumsnummer – Informationsblätter für Französischlehrer in Schule und Hochschule.* (pp. 229-233), Diesterweg, 1990.